*NEW YORK TIMES* BESTSELLER

# THE
# HORMONE
# RESET
# DIET

## HEAL YOUR METABOLISM
## TO LOSE UP TO
## 15 POUNDS IN 21 DAYS

**3**
Weeks

**7**
Hormones

**15**
Pounds

# SARA GOTTFRIED, M.D.

AUTHOR OF *THE HORMONE CURE*

FOREWORD BY MARK HYMAN, M.D.
*NEW YORK TIMES* BESTSELLING AUTHOR OF *THE BLOOD SUGAR SOLUTION*

T. Spanner

# Praise for *The Hormone Reset Diet*

"*The Hormone Reset Diet* may be just what we need to end dieting for women."
—Mark Hyman, *New York Times* bestselling author of
*The Blood Sugar Solution*

"If you're tired of storing the fat you should be burning—or simply tired of stumbling through your day—then you *need* to read this book."
—Dr. Pedram Shojai, OMD, founder of Well.org, author of
*Rise and Shine*, and producer of *Vitality*

"If you want to understand your body, you've got to start with hormones. . . Once again, Dr. Sara knocks it out of the park with this clear, user-friendly guide. "
—Jonny Bowden, Ph.D., CNS, board-certified nutritionist and
bestselling author of *The Great Cholesterol Myth*

"Science, savvy, smarts, and sexiness—it all comes together in Dr. Sara herself . . . breaking new ground in understanding how to harness our hormones, nutrition, mind, and body for optimal health."
—Mary Shomon, *New York Times* bestselling author of
*The Thyroid Diet Revolution*

"Dr. Sara Gottfried understands the extremely complex interplay between hormones, food, and environment like no one else I know."
—Jon Gabriel, bestselling author of *The Gabriel Method* and
*Visualization for Weight Loss*

"Dr. Sara Gottfried teaches you . . . that you can be guided by the innate intelligence of your female body to sustainable, peaceful balance with food and your weight."
—Jena la Flamme, author of *Pleasurable Weight Loss: The Secrets
of Feeling Great, Losing Weight, and Loving Life Today*

"Sara's new book is simple and powerful. If you have hormones, you should definitely read this book."
—Yuri Elkaim, BPHE, RHN, *New York Times* bestselling author of
*The All-Day Energy Diet*

"Sara's book is just what we need most—a woman's perspective on what it really means to feel overweight, tired, and hopeless—and a woman doctor as your guide on how to reset your entire relationship with food and yourself."
—Aviva Romm, M.D., author of *Botanical Medicine for
Women's Health*

"Dr. Sara Gottfried lays out all the reasons you feel like crap (hormones!) and how to get a handle on them [with] easy, doable advice that will save you time, energy, and money."
>                —Leanne Ely, *New York Times* bestselling author of the
>                Saving Dinner series

"Dr. Sara Gottfried's *The Hormone Reset Diet* walks you through your body's unique processes with a personalized plan for mastering your metabolism for optimal weight loss."
>                —Mark MacDonald, *New York Times* bestselling author of
>                *Body Confidence*

"Dr. Sara shares her journey of regaining her health while juggling her family's needs and a demanding career. Not only does she show that rejuvenation is possible, she gives the insights and recipes that will make it happen for you."
>                —Dr. Alan Christianson, NMD, author of *The Adrenal Reset Diet*

"I may be a man, but that doesn't mean I can't recognize the genius behind *The Hormone Reset Diet*! Every woman should have this book . . . and maybe every man, too."
>                —Abel James, author of *The Wild Diet*

"With delicious recipes and cutting-edge science, *The Hormone Reset Diet* is poised to help millions of women find the health and happiness they've been looking for."
>                —Tom Malterre, MS, CN, author of *The Elimination Diet* and
>                *The Whole Life Nutrition Cookbook*

"Occasionally a book comes along that's perfect for its time-on topic, written with authority. Such is the book by Sara Gottfried. It is a definitive integration of safe and effective approaches to the management of menopause."
>                —Jeffrey Bland, Ph.D., author of *The 20-Day Rejuvenation*
>                *Diet Program*

"Gottfried looks like an advertisement for healthy living and convincingly pushes women to make lifestyle changes rather than asking for conventional prescription drugs . . . her tips are solid and helpful."
>                —*Booklist*

"The book is both fun and an informative read [and] Gottfried's take on the female body is eye-opening and empowering."
>                —*Spirituality and Health* magazine

# THE
# HORMONE
# RESET
# DIET

HEAL YOUR METABOLISM
TO LOSE UP TO
15 POUNDS IN 21 DAYS

## SARA GOTTFRIED, M.D.

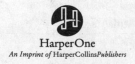

HarperOne
*An Imprint of HarperCollinsPublishers*

HarperOne

This book contains advice and information relating to health care. It should be used to supplement rather than replace the advice of your doctor or another trained health professional. If you know or suspect that you have a health problem, it is recommended that you seek your physician's advice before embarking on any medical program or treatment. All efforts have been made to assure the accuracy of the information contained in this book as of the date of publication. The publisher and the author disclaim liability for any medical outcomes that may occur as a result of applying the methods suggested in this book.

THE HORMONE RESET DIET. Copyright © 2015 by Sara Gottfried. All rights reserved. Printed in the United States of America. No part of this book may be used or reproduced in any manner whatsoever without written permission except in the case of brief quotations embodied in critical articles and reviews. For information address HarperCollins Publishers, 195 Broadway, New York, NY 10007.

HarperCollins books may be purchased for educational, business, or sales promotional use. For information please e-mail the Special Markets Department at SPsales@harpercollins.com.

HarperCollins website: http://www.harpercollins.com

FIRST HARPERCOLLINS PAPERBACK EDITION PUBLISHED IN 2016

*Designed by Terry McGrath*
*Artwork by Kevin Plottner, http://someinc.net*

Clip art throughout is from Thinkstock's iStock collection and used with permission. Images on page 41 © Kolopach, veryq, graphicsdunia4you, missbobbit, and mtkang; page 63 © Aliaksei_7799, Sergio Bellotto, and almoond; page 91 © ONiONAstudio, pavalena, and ulimi; page 108 © yuoak, ElenaNayashkova, and Cutesiness; page 117 © helgy716, Glam-Y, and Mervana; page 133 © yuoak, ElenaNayashkova, and danijelala; page 136 © olegtoka, lipmic, and ONiONAstudio; page 166 © moremarinka, ONiONAstudio, and Dynamic Graphics; page 185 © yuoak, ElenaNayashkova, and owattaphotos; page 188 © Irina_Iglina, MartinaVaculikova, and ONiONAstudio; page 208 © stolenpencil, lipmic, and ONiONAstudio; page 228 © Moriz89, fractal, and rabbitteam; pages 290–91 © Yuriy Tsirkunov.

ISBN 978–0–06–231625–7

Library of Congress Cataloging-in-Publication Data
Gottfried, Sara.
The hormone reset diet : heal your metabolism to lose up to 15 pounds in 21 days / Sara Gottfried, MD. — First edition.
    pages cm
ISBN 978–0–06–231624–0 (hardcover)
1. Weight loss. 2. Metabolism—Regulation. I. Title.
RM222.2.G68 2015
613.2'5—dc23              2014028421

16 17 18 19 20   RRD(C)   10 9 8 7 6 5 4 3

*For my beloved family,*
*David, Gemma, and Maya*

# Contents

# Foreword

The book you hold in your hands may be just what we need to end dieting for women. As I've written in my previous books, it's not your fault that you're overweight. The obesity rate has tripled in the past fifty years, and it's not because of a lack of willpower. It's because *your hormones have been hijacked by Big Food*—the giant food corporations that are similar to "Big Tobacco" and its efforts to get people addicted to cigarettes. Big Food knows how to manipulate processed food so that it's hyperpalatable and ultimately gets and keeps you addicted to these harmful food-like substances. The result is that your hormones then begin to work against you.

Enter Dr. Sara Gottfried. As a board-certified gynecologist, she is uniquely qualified to understand the private suffering that women experience with food addiction and body shame. As a Harvard-educated physician scientist, she knows how to separate good science from bad, and can translate the science into entertaining yet accurate language that everyone can understand. As a woman, she has personally struggled with and healed her own food addiction. That combination is extremely rare in medicine—few doctors are willing to admit publically their own stories of vulnerability and recovery. Not only does Dr. Sara share her stories quite poignantly, she puts them to work to change the conversation we're having about food addiction and what has been proven to solve it.

Women have specific needs compared with men and their needs are largely ignored by the $60 billion weight-loss industry that specializes in perpetuating the food lie that in order to lose weight, you must count calories.

You may have noticed that women tend to trail men when it comes to weight loss—they tend to lose weight more slowly. There are a few possible reasons for this, including:

- *Hormones.* Women have less testosterone, which boosts metabolism and keeps you lean. Men are genetically programmed to be larger and have more muscle mass and less fat. As a result, men can get away with eating more food, and when they choose to lose weight, they often get quick results.

- *Food preference.* Generally, men like meat, and women love carbohydrates—though this also may be linked to food addiction.

- *Stress.* Women tend to have more challenges with stress compared with men, according to national surveys. Their stress response system is more sensitive and vulnerable, which may explain why women are more likely to eat under emotional stress.

- *Cooking.* Women are primarily responsible for cooking the family meals. That means more work burden on women to plan menus, grocery shop, and prepare meals—plus additional temptation to taste, nibble, and lick food during cooking.

- *Dieting.* Approximately 80 percent of women are dissatisfied with their body and beat themselves up over a few extra pounds, and most are on a diet. Men are less likely to diet as a hobby. Still, there's a gender difference in expectation: women have more pressure to look like societal norms of the ideal body.

Fortunately, these gender differences can be addressed and, in many cases, turned into an advantage when you seek weight loss. Dr. Sara is here to show you how.

Remember, it's not overeating that makes you fat. It's being fat, and the hormonal chaos that led to the fat, that makes you overeat. Forget calorie counting, and begin to focus instead on the quality of your diet. This is important for both men and women, but women suffer more when it comes to food addiction, and women need a specific fix that speaks uniquely to their circumstances.

If you're a woman and having trouble with overeating, keeping your portions under control, or sugar cravings, then I highly recommend *The Hormone Reset Diet*.

I'm in constant contact with people who struggle with their weight. I've found that people often know what to do, but the problem is that most people don't have the discipline to follow through.

So instead, they fall for the tempting illusion of expensive surgeries, over-hyped exercise machines, weight loss pills, or some fad diet . . . and actually end up gaining even more weight.

Stop the madness. Recognize that food addiction has taken over your ability to modulate food, and a "cell to soul" approach is needed. Allow the wisdom of Dr. Sara and functional medicine to come to your rescue, and heal your food addiction once and for all. It's time to reset your hormones with your fork and learn to be lean naturally.

Mark Hyman, M.D.
Lenox, MA
2015

# PART ONE

# Why Women Need to Reset

# CHAPTER 1

# Women, Food, and Broken Metabolism

I used to be fat and . . . *I'm a doctor.* After decades of starving myself and feeling as though I were living in someone else's bloated body, I quit the war. In the process, I came to understand that what we've been taught about dieting is wrong—even what I was taught in medical school more than twenty-five years ago. Harsh deprivation, beating myself up over the waning willpower, daily fights with food and whether to be "good" or "bad" in my nutritional choices—these dieting skirmishes actually left me more stressed; worsened my hormonal imbalances, body shame, and food addiction; and kept me out of a genuine conversation with my body and what it actually needs.

It took me many years to learn the lesson, which occurred after trying nearly every diet, including the no-carb, low-carb, carb-cycling, low-fat, high-fat, low-protein, high-protein, no-salt, lemonade and honey, and Mediterranean diets.

The truth? These diets don't work for most women because they fail to address the hormonal root cause. Hormones dictate what your body does with food. Fatness is the result of major hormonal misfires in women, and forceful approaches to losing weight fail to address the hormonal root cause in strategy, tactics, and delivery.

Fortunately, there is a solution. You can rediscover a body you're happy with—in which you shed the weight, feel trim and sexy in your skin, and restore your hormones and health—without a daily battle. After earning a medical degree, becoming a wife, birthing two babies, and getting certified as a yoga teacher, I ultimately learned that there's an alternative to the suffering over weight that doesn't involve shame or guilt. In short, you need to correct hormonal misfires with your fork. I learned how to eat in a way that optimizes hormones and reinstates a healthy weight in women, and now I want to share my discoveries with you.

As women, we're at a disadvantage when it comes to getting fat. We are exquisitely sensitive to the ravages of stress and inflammation—you may notice the telltale signs as sugar cravings, extra weight hanging around your waist, moodiness, lack of sleep, or perhaps an overwhelmed feeling. These are clues that your hormones have begun to turn against you, which sets off a vicious cycle of inflammation (the type that makes you overweight) and more difficulty regulating the hormones that help you burn fat (also known as the hormones of metabolism, or the engine for burning calories). When misfiring hormones are allowed to spiral downward, you're left with hormone anarchy and, ultimately, a broken metabolism; and *you store fat no matter what*—even when you try popular diets like Paleo or Weight Watchers. Soon the bathroom scale seems weirdly stuck 10 or 25 pounds higher than you'd prefer. If you struggle to get and stay lean, I promise that your hormones are to blame. Your hormones govern nearly all aspects of fat loss, from where you store fat (and how much) to your cravings, appetite, gut bacteria, and even your addictive patterns with food.

The good news is that you can turn this problem around—in twenty-one days. In the pages of this book, you'll find a novel step-by-step plan that I've designed to help women of all shapes and sizes, ages and ethnicities, to lose weight and feel lighter, from your cells to your soul—a formula that has had amazing results for thousands of women just like you. I'm excited to share it with you now.

The prevailing nutritional paradigm is what I call "outside in," which refers to the hard-driving, forced march of restricting calories and maybe carbohydrates. These strategies are external and focused on physical requirements, instead of resetting your internal world and addressing the emotional issues you face. The "calories in, calories out" mind-set is the old-school approach of a one-sided conversation with the body: *You need to eat this, not that. Submit to my will.* The problem is that coercion doesn't work for women, who don't like to be forced, deprived, or disempowered. The outside-in approach tries to beat you into submission. It's a boot camp for your body, when what a woman's body really needs is three days at a spa. The female body responds far better to the coax than the shove.

## Diagnosis: Broken Metabolism

When you get a flat tire, you fix it. You don't drive around on the tire rim for ten thousand miles, ruining your car and polluting the environment. The same should be true of your metabolism. The problem is, unlike with a flat tire, sometimes you don't even know that your metabolism is broken. When it's broken, you're stuck in the fat-storage mode, depositing fat every time you eat instead of using it as fuel to energize you. When this occurs, no matter what you do—especially after age forty—you get fatter. It's not just a problem of vanity; it's as if your body is driving on a flat tire that will eventually ruin not only your metabolism but also your health if you don't repair it. Later in the process, you may develop insulin resistance (when your cells become numb to the hormone insulin) and then diabetes, heart disease, and dementia. The good news is that you *can* repair your metabolism and prevent or reverse these conditions.

When your metabolism is broken, the road to fixing it involves seven hormones that are responsible for the breakdown: estrogen, insulin, leptin, cortisol, thyroid, testosterone, and growth hormone. Each of these hormones is interconnected and interdependent with the foods you consume every day. What you are going to do is spend three short days focusing on each of these seven hormones, alone or in combination, and in a total of twenty-one days you will be fundamentally repaired and ready to turn food into energy. This is your birthright.

## Just Three Days!

The idea behind the Hormone Reset is simple: in three-day bursts, you'll focus on making specific dietary changes, starting with eliminating meat and alcohol, which resets your estrogen, liver, and gut microbiome—the genetic material of the trillions of microbial critters that live in your body. Every three days you'll cut out specific metabolism-wrecking foods and trade up for better foods, which will reset your misfiring hormones, building on the collaboration and regulatory synergy between them so you can feel like yourself again, in body harmony.

Why three days? Because that's the minimum amount of time to reset a metabolic hormone. When you disrupt these seven hormones in three-day bursts, it takes you a total of twenty-one days to recreate a collaborative team of your metabolic hormones. By the end of twenty-one days, you'll be ecstatic to observe how you feel. You'll stress less, eat clean, and move more.

## Reentry

After resetting your hormones, you'll add nutrient-dense foods back into your body, one by one, in a process called "reentry." By working with the innate intelligence of your body, you'll learn to notice, listen to, and once again *trust* your own experience when it comes to the foods that trigger your immune system into alarm mode and cause problems with weight gain. This simple strategy of adding foods back in slowly and with keen observation of your body's feedback gives you all the information you need for a future of health and vitality—based on an optimal and steady weight.

## Cell to Soul Healing

Besides making incremental dietary changes over the next twenty-one days, and beyond, we'll delve into the heart of your cravings, addictions, and habits; your ways of dealing with stress; your most deep-seated hopes and dreams for your body; and maybe even your fears and doubts about not being able to control your eating. We'll also take a bold look at how you fully inhabit your body and life.

When you're preoccupied with food, your hunger may actually be a sign of something hormonal plus something deeper. While it may suggest leptin resistance (when your cells become numb to leptin, the hormone of hunger and satiety), my opinion is that incessant hunger represents a yearning for a spiritual connection. You are experiencing a physical problem that can be solved with a combination of physical and spiritual solutions.

When you deal with the *real* issues that drive your weight gain, you don't just lose weight; you get your life back. This approach will reward you long after reaching your goal weight. I'll point you toward ways of rebuilding your confidence, integrating relaxation into your daily life, staying present, and dealing with your crazed emotions.

Many women don't have a proven structure to guide how they eat throughout the day. Usually they start off with good intentions and say confidently to themselves, "Today will be different. I'm going to be good and stop eating the refined carbs. I'll eat more vegetables. No alcohol. No sugar." But when you lack a plan that's proven to help, you end up distracted, lost, and craving the bread-basket or brownie. By six P.M., maybe you pour a glass of wine and start munching on potato chips while making dinner for your family because you're hungry for a change in your emotional state. Fast-forward a few hours, and you're heading to bed, frustrated with yourself and your body. You feel a lack of integrity with your stated aspiration for how you want to look, eat, and live. Further, it's really hard to break through—and get the lean body you want—because you get stuck in this destructive cycle. At the end of the day, perhaps you say to yourself, "Darn it! I didn't do what I wanted with food yet again. I failed myself. There's another day lost."

I don't want this frustration to sweep over you another day. If you follow my plan, you won't have a single day of going to bed exasperated with yourself and your lack of willpower. You'll experience something far better. This plan has worked for thousands of women who have felt hopeless, scared, ashamed, and unlovable—and it can work for you too.

Remind yourself from this day on that working from the inside out (instead of outside in) takes time, which in my experience is a minimum of twenty-one days. I'll be your guide along the road. You'll also be empowered to become the ultimate authority on the best foods for you.

With the Hormone Reset you'll learn how to

- reset your weight, nutrition, hormones, and habitual patterns, from cell to soul;
- build new habits that keep you from depending on willpower;
- become rewired to self-care;
- approach the process as a new devotion, not a slog;
- close the gap between your intention and your behavior; and
- stay present to the here and now of your relationship to food—the good, the bad, and the ugly—because otherwise you may miss a sacred opportunity to learn more about yourself, the effect food is having on your hormones, and how you use food beyond mere sustenance.

I know you've been promised solutions before and you may feel hopeless. This time is different because I have thousands of case studies from all types of women that prove resetting metabolic hormones works. I'm asking you to trust me until you can see it for yourself.

Your body is sending you divine messages that desire to be decoded, understood, processed, and assimilated. Listen. Your body is not lying to you. When you trust the signals from your body as truth and allow them to guide your choices, you become like a windmill that generates renewable and clean energy for the power grid. It's an alchemical shift when you get lean from cell to soul, and I've learned—as a seasoned gynecologist and scientist—that there is unlimited potential for you to feel brimming with energy, fun, and passion when you truly understand how to nourish the female body. I have one word to describe it: grace.

As you may know, grace does not easily coexist with chronic stress, a muffin top, or high blood sugar. When you reconstitute internally and change your ecosystem, you transform externally, and it's palpable. You'll look, feel, and become biologically younger. There's a bounce in your step. You switch to the "lean" position instead of the "fat" position. Obstacles to weight loss melt away. Loving people are attracted to you. You know the type I'm referring to: the people who make you feel more fully yourself.

If you don't heed the call your body is sending to you—in the form of weight gain, belly fat, fatigue, and feeling old before your time—there may be repercussions. A subtle biochemical downshift may take over your body, showing up as food addiction, shame, regret, prediabetes, chronic pain, autoimmune conditions, depression, grief, and the deepest sadness of what might have been. Why wait? The Hormone Reset asks you to evolve in two essential ways: to eat in a way that is aligned with your female genetics (the cellular method) and to integrate the physical aspects of this food plan with your psychology and spirituality (the soul method).

You can no longer afford merely to go through the motions of living: the dysfunction in your work, the porous boundaries with your kids and work, the ailing relationship with your partner, the lack of meaning in your job, or the high-stress lifestyle that has taken over your life. It's time to turn your struggles around with a feeling of certainty about your body and future. Most of our beliefs are generalizations about our past, based on painful experiences and a lack of success. Many of us don't decide in a fully conscious and empowered way what to believe, and we get stuck with beliefs that are limiting and unnecessarily constricting. Over the next three weeks, we will take on these limiting beliefs and habitual patterns, and swap them for something far better. I did it, and you can too.

## My Big Fat Story

Like many of you, I have struggled to be lean most of my life. I feel fortunate that through circumstance—combined with luck and the application of my medical knowledge—my struggle with weight and food ended when I was in my thirties.

I first gained weight when I was about ten years old. I craved sugar, especially my grandmother's chocolate chip cookie dough. My grandmother told me that the dough contained raw eggs so I shouldn't eat it. But I didn't listen. It's my first memory of considering an adult's opinion about nutrition and dismissing it in favor of the taste of food. Taste trumped wisdom. I wanted to stop but couldn't. In that moment, I became a food addict.

When I was fifteen, I started restricting food and calories, longing to be thin and to look cute in my jeans. I'd starve myself all day, relying on willpower and diet soda (remember Tab?), and end up bingeing on freshly baked chocolate chip cookies or sugary pastries. In my freshman year of college, I ballooned to 150 pounds (I'm five feet, five inches tall). That summer I started running and drinking bee pollen smoothies, and lo and behold, I was 125 pounds by the start of sophomore year. Every time I had a new boyfriend, I would eat like he did and gain weight. I would be fat and happy. Then our breakup would lead to a loss of appetite. I would become thin and sad.

My weight came into sharp focus when I got engaged. I had six months until my wedding day to get thin. The Atkins diet was popular at the time, so my fiancé, David Gottfried, and I started eating more eggs and bacon, and "Please hold the toast!" David dropped 20 pounds, and I dropped 2. I stared at my tight wedding dress in frustration. As a gynecologist who was board certified in everything that goes wrong in the female body, I knew something was amiss. I filed my observations away and went on with my wedding preparations, forcing myself to lose weight with willpower, calorie restriction, and overexercising, like a drill sergeant determined to fit into my wedding dress. I became an uptight, slightly thinner bride. But I gained the weight back within a single week during our honeymoon in Hawaii!

In my thirties, I spent way too much of my time and brain obsessing over food and how to restrict it. I was a working mom. I plugged away during the day as a busy doctor and came home for a second shift of childcare and preparing a meal for my family. I felt a large void in my life, probably because I found the idea of "having it all" ridiculously impossible and exhausting, and I didn't realize that I was trying to fill that void with refined carbohydrates and glasses of wine. I was stressed, fat, toxic, unhappy, resentful, and inflamed— and nothing seemed to help. Even my blood sugar suffered: tests showed levels consistent with early diabetes.

My defining moment came in an unlikely setting: a Madonna concert. As she sang and danced for more than two hours, I was moved by her physical majesty, by the grace of how fully she embodied her feminine power. I had a flash of insight. Did I want to reach my highest potential? Or did I want to keep making excuses and stay on the downward spiral of getting fatter, more burned out, and further from my inner vision of greatness? It was one of those moments of deep clarity—some even call them surrender points—that addicts talk about, when the pain of staying the same comes into sharp relief. I decided that it was time to take action and to apply my medical knowledge to help myself.

The next day I joined a program for food addicts. I wasn't an obese, bingeing type of addict. I was highly functional and looked relatively "normal" from the outside. Still, there was an obsessive quality to food and eating that kept me hooked, especially during high stress.

I learned more about women, food, and the importance of a spiritual solution in that program than I had ever learned in medical school. Within two months, I lost 25 pounds, reset my hormones and blood sugar, and healed my broken metabolism. I stayed in the program for two years—stable at the same weight, week after week— but eventually left for several reasons. The program didn't seem to help my other hormone issues, such as with thyroid and estrogen. In fact, some of the food rules seemed old-school and failed to address important nutritional gaps. Ultimately, I was motivated to learn how to help myself and all women calibrate their hormones and, by extension, their metabolisms without having to surrender to the rigid structure of a program with regular meetings.

Here's what led to the book you have in your hands:

- I took my deep knowledge of the female body from the past twenty years as a board-certified gynecologist and physician-scientist;

- I studied the latest advances in our understanding of food addiction, since this piece is often missing from popular diets and disproportionately affects women;

- I combined the best practices from my experience in the food addiction program and removed the parts that didn't seem necessary to my recovery;

- I learned why women eat for a state change—also known as emotional eating—and developed effective alternatives;
- I added extensive and current research about hormone imbalances, resets, and detoxification;
- I interviewed world experts on hormones, introduced novel information about gender differences in fatness and how women can turn vulnerabilities into advantages in the battle of the bulge; and finally,
- I turned it all into my own personal plan, culled from my knowledge based on twenty years of medical practice, which has worked for me and now works for thousands of other women like you.

I taught the Hormone Reset program for the first time in 2008 to a group of women in my integrative and functional medicine practice in Oakland, California. The process and synthesis showed me the key steps that women need to take to break the shackles of food addiction, heal emotionally, form new habits of eating the best types and quantities of nourishing food, and recalibrate to eating for the right reasons. The results were transformative: The women felt at home in their bodies again and were excited to repeat the program every three to six months with me. They described many of the feelings that I experienced myself. Consistently, they lost weight—about 10 to 50 pounds—and they told me they felt younger than they did ten or twenty years ago.

I've tested, honed, and improved my Hormone Reset program in my medical practice, my in-person group programs, and online for the past six years. In this book, you now have access to the same wildly successful twenty-one-day weight-loss program. You have everything you need to break the addictive cycle of eating the wrong foods, stressing, and feeling fat once and for all. With it, you can restore your broken, overstressed body and find the grace and magnificence promised you by the wonders of your own unique biology.

# CHAPTER 2

# Prep for Your Hormone Reset

It's time to lay the foundation for your Hormone Reset. Preparation is behind every lasting change when it comes to your body and losing weight for good. Otherwise, modernity conspires against you such that your nervous system is toast, you feel overwhelmed and poisoned by hormones, and you are at the mercy of food cravings. I've found the best antidote is intention, so I've created a plan for you to prioritize space for the sacred—in your head, heart, and schedule—in the day or two before starting your Hormone Reset.

The preparation phase is a time of emotional, physical, and spiritual arrangements, if you allow it to be. It takes planning to connect to your inner divinity so that it may guide you to your cure. Setting the right intention will create the ideal vibrational tone for the body to begin to reset hormones, release weight and toxins, and heal addictive patterns. You have nothing to lose (except weight, of course!) and everything to gain. On your mark, get set . . . *prepare*!

# Self-Assessment

Does your weight keep you from living your biggest, fullest, richest life? Do you suffer from food addiction? Are you a stress case? *Welcome to the club!* You are in the right place, because we are going to fix these issues, starting immediately. Take the following self-assessment to find out if you need the Hormone Reset. In the past six months, have you experienced . . .

☐ Looking in the mirror and not liking what you see?

☐ Limiting certain activities until you finally lose the weight, such as sex or going to the beach?

☐ Eating or craving certain foods, even when you're not hungry? Snacking all day? Observing that you get hungry not long after eating a meal (i.e., within less than four hours)?

☐ Noticing that your weight seems to fluctuate constantly?

☐ Jumping from one diet to another, looking for the magic bullet? Occasionally restricting your food, though you're able to sustain this only a short while?

☐ Feeling tired or sluggish after eating?

☐ Hiding food or eating in secrecy? Keeping a secret stash of chocolate or sweets in your special drawer or cabinet?

☐ Weighing yourself every day? Being in either a good or a bad mood for the day depending on the number on the bathroom scale?

☐ Eating more than you planned or bingeing? Noticing that you have avalanche foods: you take one bite, and shortly thereafter, the whole container is gone? Feeling guilty about how much (quantity) or the types of food (quality) you're eating? Eating until you feel uncomfortably full?

☐ Purging? Overeating and then taking a laxative, vomiting, or exercising to make up for it?

☐ Experiencing health issues from overeating—including diagnoses from your doctor, such as prediabetes, diabetes, high cholesterol, metabolic syndrome—or just being told you need to lose weight to get healthier?

☐ Observing that you need more of certain foods for them to bring you the same pleasure as they used to provide, such as chocolate, wine, or french fries?

☐ Thinking about your weight or food constantly?

☐ Continuing to eat foods that have negative consequences for you, such as weight gain, bloating, belly pain, gas, or other signs that the foods don't agree with your body?

### Interpret Your Results

- **If you have five or more of these indicators,** you are so ready for the Hormone Reset that you can come straight through the starting gate now! Food, stress, and negative habits have handcuffed you, as noted from the self-assessment (adapted with significant changes for my patients from the Yale Food Addiction Scale, which has been validated in women).[1] Together, we are going to remove the cuffs and get you back to an empowered, healthy version of yourself.

- **If you have four or fewer of these symptoms or are unsure,** you may be teetering on the edge of food addiction and unhealthy eating. I want you to come back to solid ground before it's too late! I heartily recommend that you start your Hormone Reset to prevent food issues from later causing more weight gain and health problems.

## Overview of Your Hormone Reset

In your Hormone Reset we will resynchronize the seven hormones of metabolism. Here is the order of hormone resets that I've found to be the most effective:

1. *Meatless,* designed to reset your estrogen by excluding red meat and alcohol from your diet. (Note that this reset is essential for everyone, whether you're a meat eater or not.)

2. *Sugar Free,* intended to banish your cravings for sugar and reset your insulin.

3. *Fruitless,* targeted to reset your hunger hormone, leptin.

4. *Caffeine Free,* which will reset your relationship to stress and cortisol.

5. *Grain Free,* formulated to activate your thyroid hormone in a powerful new way and will reset insulin and leptin.

6. *Dairy Free,* designed to reset your growth hormone, which also improves insulin.

7. *Toxin Free,* which will redirect your testosterone level to normal, along with supporting the reset of estrogen, insulin, leptin, and thyroid.

After you take all these steps, you will have reset your metabolism.

I'm so excited for you because you're about to enter the circle of hormone resets (as shown in the following figure) that expedite major body transformation from the inside out. I know what it's like at the top, after completing the first round of seven hormone resets—I can see the comprehensive view from here, and it's amazing. Yes, you will fix your broken metabolism and lose weight. But more important, you will take the crucial steps you need to feel at home in your body again. You will break the relentless cycle of stress and weight gain. You won't be constantly bloated, stressed, or sleep deprived. You will grow the happy and diverse bacteria that keep you lean and shed the bacteria that make you fat.

Reaching these goals begins with awareness and preparation. Don't worry; you aren't alone. I will hold your hand through every step of the way. In this chapter, you'll find everything you need to enter the circle starting first with the estrogen reset, including a checklist, a shopping guide, baseline measurements, and key action steps to activate your Hormone Reset.

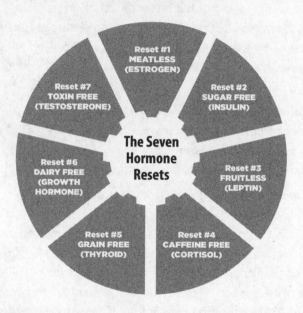

## Checklist

In order to set you up for success with the first reset, review these high-priority items. If you're feeling overwhelmed, just focus on completing what is required for the first reset. If you're feeling generally okay with your preparations and in the mood for extra credit, add some or all of the optional items.

### Required

☐ **Choose your Day 1.** This is the start day of the twenty-one-day Hormone Reset. Many women choose Monday, but it's your body and your decision.

☐ **Buy a small journal.** Make sure it fits into your purse or on your nightstand. Make it pretty. You'll be committing to your food each night for the next day, thereby setting up a sense of integrity and accomplishment when you eat the foods you've planned. You'll be archiving your thoughts, feelings, wins, and challenges as you progress through your Hormone Reset—not merely as a recording of events but rather as a clarifying tool that helps you know yourself, solve problems, and release old emotions. Journaling is essential to clean eating and recovery, and science proves that it helps boost cognitive function, counteracts stress, and bolsters immunity.

☐ **Collect the first four of the ten recommended measurements (on the tracker, page 26).** Note that if you want the best results, I recommend you perform all ten measurements prior to starting the program.

☐ **Clear the decks.** Remove from your pantry, refrigerator, and freezer the food culprits that commonly cause hormonal misfires: alcohol, red meats, sugar, sugar substitutes, sodas and diet sodas, coffee and other caffeinated beverages, high-fructose fruits, grains (including gluten), and dairy products. Enlist your family to support or even join your journey to improve your health, since they will benefit from it too, even if they don't have weight to lose. If you don't live alone or your family declines to join you in clearing the decks, create special shelves in the pantry, refrigerator, and freezer—not at eye level so you're not tempted—where you store these foods for others in the household.

☐ **Copy the shopping lists (or photograph them with your smartphone).** Using the shopping lists provided later in this chapter (page 34), go to the store and, at a minimum, buy everything for the first reset, Meatless. You will be off red meat and need clean protein alternatives.

☐ *Take a quick "before" picture.* Snap a selfie, or ask someone to take photos of the front, each side, and back of your body before you begin.

## Optional

☐ *Perform additional measurements.* The more you objectively measure and track the progress of your blood pressure, body fat, blood sugar, and waist and hip circumferences, the more you will improve. If you initially chose to take just the first four of the ten measurements, add a few more from the tracker (page 26).

☐ *Solicit a friend to join you.* Find an accountability partner! I know that people who perform programs like this one together lose twice as much weight.

☐ *Purchase supplements:*

   ☐ *Shake powder.* When you are shifting the way that you eat, you can make life simpler by substituting a shake for a meal. This practice is optional, but I find that shakes provide the essential ingredients you need to reset your hormones, detoxify, and fill nutrient gaps. If you want to eat only food and to drink only filtered water, no problem; plenty of women have succeeded on the Hormone Reset without shakes. If you want shakes as an option, purchase a nondairy, nonwhey protein powder. I recommend that you follow my program to the letter, which means you need to obtain enough shake powder for at least thirty-six servings. (See Resources for my favorite shake powders.) Here are several nutritional requirements that work well for people who have completed my program successfully (check the label of the shake, and make sure you have the following per serving):

   • Protein: 15 grams (minimum), but 20 grams is preferred
   • Maximum net carbs (total carbs less total fiber): 8 grams, but less is preferred

- Maximum sugar: 5 grams, but less is preferred

☐ **Fiber.** As you will find during the first reset, fiber helps you activate estrogen so it's in the fat-burning zone. Order or pick up from your local health food store a fiber blend, at least thirty-six servings' worth. You want to find the type of fiber that keeps you pooping and doesn't cause constipation. The average woman in the United States consumes 12 to 14 grams of fiber per day. Plan to gradually increase your fiber intake by a maximum of 5 grams per day so that your body can adjust. For example, aim for 17 grams on Day 1, 22 grams on Day 2, 27 grams on Day 3, etc., until you are consuming 35 to 45 grams per day.

☐ **Consult a health professional before getting started.** If you have or suspect that you have any serious health conditions, including but not limited to diabetes or high blood pressure, and/or if you take any medications, talk to your doctor. Although this program is gradual and gentle, and it has been completed by thousands of women, it's important to know that some people experience significant reductions in blood sugar and blood pressure.

☐ **Baseline laboratory tests.** Throughout your Hormone Reset, you will find my recommendations for tests that you can order yourself or request from your health professional. These are optional but may elucidate which of your hormones are misfiring.

## The Writing Cure

Ready for your first assignment? Break out that pretty new journal, and we'll begin. The first question to answer in your journal is an important one that will set your long-term vision for yourself: What will it feel like to be at home in your body?

We are each so unique, with our own history, perspective, and opinions. I asked women who had completed the Hormone Reset about being at home in their bodies, and here are a few of their answers:

> "To be comfortable with who I am and have that sense of fulfillment that I'm living in my ultimate purpose, in the healthiest way—body, soul, and spirit. It's knowing where I've been, where I am in the present, and where I'm heading for eternity!" —*Katie*

> "To be home in my body would be the feeling of peace and balance. No pain, no extra 'stuffing' in the wrong places, calm and relaxed and fully functioning body." —*Monica*

## APPLYING THE ORGANIZATIONAL CHANGE MODEL

Almost all of us know the basics about what to do to lose weight and feel healthy. When we follow a healthy eating plan, we feel great and vow to keep at it. But alas, human nature is complex. Even the best intentioned of us find it hard to sustain that plan.

I struggle with this problem myself. As a scientist, I went to my default: research. This led me to study the burgeoning field of change management so I could apply the best practices to my own life and then teach them to the women who work with me online and in my medical practice. Change management is an approach that helps people or groups move from the current state to a desired future state. The latest research tells us that we need to apply the following when going through a change:

**Set a big vision.** For instance, "I want to lose 25 pounds" or "I want to bring my fasting blood sugar from the prediabetes range of 110 mg/dL down to the normal range of 70 to 85" or "I'm committing to implementing seven resets in twenty-one days."

**Break the big vision into smaller goals that you can easily achieve.** *Try saying to yourself, "Today, I am resetting my insulin resistance. I will stay on task with my insulin reset for three days and then move to the next module, which is to banish fructose and reset my leptin" or "I'm committing to writing my next day's food every evening."*

**Rise above the fray.** *Don't get caught up with the minutiae. Stick to the big vision and your smaller goals. Write your goals on Post-its and keep them handy so that they trigger your intention: place the Post-its on your bathroom mirror, in your wallet, on your refrigerator, on the steering wheel in your car. If you slip up, be gentle with yourself. I use my smartphone to take a picture of my big vision and smaller goals, and I use the image as the wallpaper on my smartphone, so every time I unlock my phone, I see it and connect to my intention.*

*Change can feel intimidating, and sometimes you may find yourself momentarily resisting your big vision and/or your smaller goals. Remind yourself that these moments will pass. If you're feeling overwhelmed, focus on the first three-day reset. Be sweet to yourself and keep moving forward—even small steps that feel inconsequential add up to major transformation over time.*

---

## Your Top Ten Measurements

One of the most important aspects of your Hormone Reset is measuring your results. This will help you capture a snapshot of your current health as well as the progress you make during the course of this program. I find it helps to set small goals for specific outcomes beyond losing weight. What you measure improves and connects you to intention—that is, it's harder to change something you're unaware of, such as your body fat.

The following is a list of the top ten measurements I recommend you take before, during, and after your Hormone Reset, to track your progress. Measurements one through four are mandatory; they are easy and require very few supplies. Measurements five through ten are highly recommended but optional. (For additional information, see Resources.)

## Measurement #1: Waist and Hips

**Frequency:** Before Day 1 and weekly
**Supplies Needed:** A soft tape measure
**Instructions:** Measure your waist circumference, at your belly button and also one inch above your belly button. Make sure the tape measure is not too tight and that it's parallel with the floor. Don't hold your breath while measuring! Write down your measurements in inches or centimeters. You will use the measurement at your belly button to calculate your waist-to-hip ratio and the measurement one inch above your belly button for your waist-to-height ratio.

Also measure your hips—the circumference of your hips at the widest point. Try to use a similar degree of snugness each time you measure. Then calculate the waist-to-hip ratio by dividing your waist measurement by your hip measurement, or go to www.health calculators.org.[2]

Which shape are you? Indicate your measurements in the tracker or cut and paste into your journal. For all the possible waist-to-hip ratios and what they mean for women, see the following breakdown.

# The Hormone Reset Tracker

|  | Before Day 1 | Day 22 |
|---|---|---|
|  | Date | Date |
| Waist (inches or centimeters) | _____ | _____ |
| Hip (inches or centimeters) | _____ | _____ |
| Waist-to-hip ratio | _____ | _____ |
| Weight (pounds or kilograms) | _____ | _____ |
| Height (inches or meters) | _____ | _____ |
| Basal Metabolic Rate | _____ | _____ |
| Hormones (My Hormone Score™) | _____ | _____ |
| Body mass index | _____ | _____ |
| Waist-to-height ratio | _____ | _____ |
| Sleep (total hours or score) | _____ | _____ |
| Blood pressure (mm Hg) | _____ | _____ |
| Blood sugar (mg/dL) | _____ | _____ |
| Steps (total per day) | _____ | _____ |
| Body fat (percent) | _____ | _____ |
| Carbohydrates (total grams per day) | _____ | _____ |
| Fiber (total grams per day) | _____ | _____ |
| Net carbohydrates (grams) | _____ | _____ |
| pH | _____ | _____ |

- *A waist-to-hip ratio of 0.80 or less.* You are a "pear" shape and at low risk of health problems. Good job! You may still have a broken metabolism, and together we will work to get your ratio even better.

- *A waist-to-hip ratio of 0.81 to 0.85.* You are an "avocado" shape and are at moderate risk of health issues. The Hormone Reset is designed to improve your waist-to-hip ratio over the next twenty-one days, and hopefully—if you follow the plan carefully—you will reduce your risk by lowering your ratio.

- *A waist-to-hip ratio of 0.86 or higher.* You are an "apple" shape, and you are at increased risk of blood sugar problems, prediabetes, diabetes, stroke, heart disease, metabolic syndrome, and hip fractures. You would benefit from performing all ten measurements and following the Hormone Reset closely.

## Measurement #2: Body Mass Index, Waist-to-Height Ratio, and Basal Metabolic Rate

**Frequency:** Before Day 1 and the first day of each reset

**Supplies Needed:** A bathroom scale, a yardstick or tape measure to measure your most recent height accurately, and a computer with Internet access

**Instructions:** Always weigh yourself first thing in the morning, before eating breakfast. Write down your weight in pounds or kilograms.

Also determine your height. As a population, we shrink as we age from poor posture and osteoporosis, so please get an accurate height, either at home or when you go to see your practitioner prior to starting the Hormone Reset. Write it down in inches or centimeters.

From your accurate preprogram height and weight measurements, you can calculate important metrics for your tracker:

- *Body mass index (BMI).* Use an online calculator or the formula (BMI = weight ÷ height$^2$).[3] If you use kilograms and centimeters, you have your result. If you use pounds and inches, you need to multiply the result by 703. (See Notes for more details and examples.[4]) For example, for a woman who is 150 pounds with a height of five feet four inches (64 inches total),

$$\text{BMI} = (150 \div 64^2) \times 703 = 25.7$$

- *Waist-to-height ratio (WHtR).* One recent study of 3,937 women in the United Kingdom showed that their waist-to-height ratio predicted their risk of diabetes better than their BMI. Other studies concur.[5] To calculate your WHtR, take your waist measurement from measurement one (one inch above your belly button) and divide that by your height in inches (or use an online calculator[6]). If you're female, keep your WHtR less than 0.49. If your WHtR is 0.50 or higher, let's work together to get the ratio down over the next twenty-one days.

- *Basal metabolic rate (BMR).* Your BMR is the amount of calories that you burn at rest over twenty-four hours (if you stayed in bed all day). The result helps you determine whether your metabolism is fast or slow. You can measure it at a gym (usually as a resting metabolic rate, based on the oxygen you inhale and the carbon dioxide you exhale), or you can calculate an estimate based on your weight, height, and age. Use an online calculator (see Resources) or the following formula if you can't make it to a participating gym.

$$\text{BMR} = 655 + (4.35 \times \text{weight in pounds}) + (4.7 \times \text{height in inches}) - (4.7 \times \text{age})$$

Continuing with our example of a woman who is 150 pounds with a height of five feet four inches, and an age of forty,

$$\text{BMR} = 655 + (4.35 \times 150) + (4.7 \times 64) - (4.7 \times 40) = 1420$$

Once you know your BMR, you can determine your daily caloric burn by adjusting BMR based on your physical fitness. For someone who exercises lightly one to three days per week, you multiple BMR by 1.375. Sedentary folks use BMR × 1.2, and people who moderately exercise three to five times per week, use BMR × 1.55.

In our example, our 150-pound woman walks for thirty minutes three times per week, so her daily caloric need is approximately 1420 × 1.375 = 1953 calories per day. While weight loss is not simply a matter of calories in and calories out, BMR can give you a ballpark for where your metabolism is at the beginning and end of the program. You can raise your BMR by resetting your metabolic hormones, lifting weights, and burst training.

## Measurement #3: Hormones

**Frequency:** Before Day 1 and again on Day 22

**Supplies Needed:** A computer with Internet access or *The Hormone Cure*

**Instructions:** My Hormone Score is a quiz that has been formulated to help you quickly identify which of your hormones and neurotransmitters are imbalanced. You can take the online assessment at www.thehormonecurebook.com/quiz/ or purchase my book, *The Hormone Cure,* for the full-length version. If you use the full-length version, tally the total number of "yes" answers for each hormone imbalance and record that number as your score on your tracker (page 26). If you're using the online quiz, make a note in your journal of which hormones may be out of balance prior to starting your Hormone Reset, and you can revisit the quiz again after you've completed the twenty-one days.

## Measurement #4: Sleep

**Frequency:** Daily

**Supplies Needed:** Nothing is needed to measure total sleep; use a sleep tracking device to measure type of sleep (see my recommendations in the Shopping Guide, page 34).

**Instructions:** At a minimum, you should record the quantity and quality of your sleep each night using a journal. Better yet would be to measure your type of sleep using a tracking device. On the Jawbone UP device, for example, you will receive a "sleep score" each night or a percentage of ideal sleep for you based on your age and sleep patterns. If you're using the UP, record your Day 0 sleep score from the main app page on your smartphone.

## Measurement #5: Blood Pressure

**Frequency:** Before Day 1 and again on Day 22 or later

**Supplies Needed:** You can measure your blood pressure at home, at your practitioner's office, or at your local drugstore.

**Instructions:** There are two important numbers to pay attention to when you measure your blood pressure. The top number is called your "systolic" blood pressure, and it should be less than 140 mm Hg (millimeters of mercury). The bottom number is called your "diastolic" blood pressure, and it should be less than 90 mm Hg.

## Measurement #6: Blood Sugar

**Frequency:** Daily; however, measure every three days if your fasting and postprandial (after a meal) blood sugar levels are in the optimal ranges.

**Supplies Needed:** A blood glucose meter (you can purchase one at your local drugstore without a prescription), blood glucose test strips, a lancing device, lancets, and a control solution (optional)

**Instructions:** There are two important times to check your blood sugar. The first is in the morning after you've not eaten for eight to twelve hours, and the second is two hours after you've eaten. Start by measuring your fasting blood sugar before eating breakfast. In addition, it's helpful to measure your blood sugar two hours after a meal, particularly dinner.

I provide a detailed, step-by-step description of how to do this on my website,[7] or have someone at your doctor's office teach you how to do it.

## Measurement #7: Steps

**Frequency:** Daily

**Supplies Needed:** A step-tracking device or a pedometer (see my recommendations in the Shopping Guide, page 34)

**Instructions:** Adaptive and moderate exercise is very important during the Hormone Reset, because it can speed the release of toxins and heal your metabolism. Tracking your total steps per day will help you monitor and increase your daily activity.

## Measurement #8: Body Fat

**Frequency:** Before Day 1 and again on Day 22

**Supplies Needed:** A special body fat scale (see Resources) or caliper measurements or bioelectrical impedance analysis at your local gym

**Instructions:** It's easy to get fixated on the number on your bathroom scale, but body fat can be a much more accurate indicator of health and fitness. Your body is a complex combination of fluid, bone, muscle, and fat; a single number on a scale isn't sufficient to capture your progress on this program.

The most accurate measurement of fat is with bioelectrical imped-ance analysis (BIA), which can be done for fifteen dollars at my local university, for example. Search "BOD POD" online to see if there's a device near you where you can accurately measure your body fat.

## Measurement #9: Net Carbohydrates

**Frequency:** Daily

**Supplies Needed:** None, or a simple calculator (such as on your phone) or app

**Instructions:** Your goal from Day 1 through Day 21 is to keep your net carbohydrates at between 20 to 49 grams per day. Net carbs are calculated by determining your total carbohydrate intake (in grams) and deducting the total fiber intake (in grams). For instance, I aim to keep my total carbohydrates at approximately 75 grams per day when I'm trying to lose weight and 100 to 150 grams when I'm maintaining my weight. I eat 35 to 45 grams of fiber per day. If each day, from Day 1 through Day 21, I eat 75 grams of carbohydrates and 40 grams of fiber, my daily net carbs are 35 grams (75–40 = 35). Record your net carbs before Day 1 on your tracker (page 26) so you get the hang of it.

## Measurement #10: pH

**Frequency:** Daily; every three days if your pH level is over 7.0 consistently

**Supplies Needed:** pH test strips

**Instructions:** I recommend testing the pH of your urine first thing in the morning. Instructions are typically included with the test strips and generally consist of letting some of your urine hit the test strip mid-stream, waiting a few moments, and then comparing the color of the test strip to the colors on the package to find out your current pH level. Your pH level is an important measure of overall health (see page 178).

## Gently Shifting Your Habits

How many times do you really think about brushing your teeth? My guess is not many. It's just something you do, even if you don't want to. You don't rely on willpower, because it's a habit. Part of the reason for your acceptance is that you've been doing it for a long time. You know that if you don't, you might suffer the consequences.

I want to make eating healthy food and sustaining your ideal weight as easy as brushing your teeth, which will require creating new habits. Before you become overwhelmed by this task, let's break it down. You can do this. You might be surprised at how easy creating new habits becomes once you enjoy the benefits of weight loss, increased energy, and fewer mood swings. Choose one or more of the following actions to create new habits in the next three days:

- *Write.* Start writing in your Hormone Reset journal. Why do you want to be healthy? I believe healthy people have more fun and true connection with others—but that's me.

- *Listen.* Tune in to your body before you act. This could mean acting on an impulse to eat or reacting to your child's whining. Tune in, listen, and identify the feelings in your body. Do you feel an ache in your belly? A tightening in your chest? Is your breathing restricted or full? Simply noticing your bodily sensations will help you identify your feelings and think before you act.

- *Notice.* Pay attention to your life energy. What makes it strong, and what makes it weak? What stops it from flowing? Write the answers in your journal and see where your writing leads and what insights it provides.

## Get Ready to . . . Reset!

Over the next twenty-one days you will gradually eliminate the foods and reset the seven hormones that are most likely slowing down your metabolism. If that feels daunting, don't fret. I've included here a shopping guide and grocery lists to set you up for success.

What you eat affects your body, mind, and spirit far more than simply interacting with your taste buds. Food is intimate. When it's carefully chosen for nutritional value to your specific body, it is assimilated swiftly and easily, and it builds who you are, cell by cell. Think about how you feel the morning after a heavy meal or too much to drink. Consider your mood after you eat a lot of sugar or drink loads of coffee. As you prepare to buy your food for the first reset of your Hormone Reset, hit the pause button and consider what you've been filling yourself with up to this point and my recommended replacements. The goal is to become far more mindful of the type of person you want to become—a happy, content, and whole individual with a rich inner and outer life. You can begin to create this, starting with how you eat.

## Shopping Guide

Preparation is key to your success. The following shopping lists are just a starting point to help you get a feel for your options at the grocery store; there are plenty of wonderful foods not on these lists. Feel free to select only the items you like, or go on an adventure and search out healthy items that you haven't yet tried.

### SHOPPING RULES OF THUMB

*Buy organic whenever possible.*

*Buy fresh, unprocessed foods.*

*Aim to eat one pound of vegetables per day! Get creative with different salads and recipes.*

*Buy local.* Farmers' markets are a great place to get fresh, local food. Just be sure to ask where the food was grown/made. Don't assume it's local or organic just because you bought it at a farmers' market!

*Buy non-GM (genetically modified) foods.* I believe it's your right as a consumer to know what's in your food, including GMs. Your safest bet is to check the listings at the Non-GMO Project, which verifies non-GM foods.[8] Another option is to choose organic foods, which do not contain GMOs. Fortunately, grassroots efforts across the United States indicate that citizens want to know what's in their food: twenty-nine states now have bills for GMO labeling.[9] The nine most common GM crops are soy, cottonseed (used for fabric and oil), corn, canola oil, papaya, alfalfa, sugar beets (used to produce half the sugar in the United States), milk (17 percent of U.S. dairy cows are injected with recombinant bovine growth hormone, or rBGH, a genetically modified synthetic hormone), and aspartame (an artificial sweetener commonly used in diet soda as well as six thousand other products; it's also known as NutraSweet).

*Read labels,* making sure you understand what the ingredients really are. Dairy, sugar, gluten, and other substances can be hidden under different names. If you're not certain, Google the ingredient you don't recognize or just skip that food.

*Bring your own bags.* The Hormone Reset is an important opportunity to explore different ways of leading a more healthy and environmentally conscious lifestyle. Bringing reusable bags to the grocery store is a small step that can really add up over time.

*Embrace your inner chef.* Making food from scratch is one of the best ways to ensure you know exactly what you're eating. Set aside time to cook and experiment in the kitchen each week. You might be surprised how much you enjoy it!

*Make extra,* and take the leftovers for lunch. While the ideal is always to make your food fresh, the reality is that most of us get too *busy. When you do have time to cook, make extra so that you can re-heat or repurpose it for other meals later (especially staples like clean protein and vegetables).*

---

## Nonfood Items

- ☐ **Blender.** If you want to splurge on an amazing blender that will last, I recommend the Vitamix or the Blendtec. A less expensive version that still gets you the fiber you need and travels more easily is the NutriBullet. However, any blender will do the job. (You can also use a shaker bottle for travel.)

- ☐ **Food scale.** Use a food scale daily to keep your food portions accurate. This tool is particularly important for food addicts, who may have lost their judgment on portion size.

- ☐ **Blood glucose meter.** Testing your blood sugar can be one of the most valuable aspects of this program because it will dramatically increase your awareness of how certain foods affect your body.

- ☐ **pH test strips.** Test your urine pH with these strips to assess how acid or alkaline your body is and how food impacts your pH. Buy at least thirty strips to last through Reentry.

- ☐ **Soft tape measure.** You'll need this to take your initial measurements and to track your slimming waist and hip circumferences.

- ☐ **Bathroom scale and/or body fat scale.** Weigh yourself at the beginning of each reset. You can also purchase a body fat scale or visit your local gym to get your body fat measurement taken.

- ☐ **Sleep and step trackers.** I recommend the UP by Jawbone to track both your sleep and your total steps per day (as well as your food, with the convenient app) because it's essentially all in one. Alternatives for tracking your sleep include the Basis, the Lark, and the Fitbit. Alternatives for tracking your total steps include the Nike+ FuelBand, Fitbit, iPhone, and a regular pedometer.

☐ **Dry brush.** One of the daily rituals I suggest integrating during your Hormone Reset is dry brushing your skin and stimulating your lymphatic system before you bathe in the morning. This practice can be an invigorating replacement for your morning cup of caffeine. The technique is to brush your dry and naked skin, head to toe or toe to head. Long strokes across your skin exfoliate best: from the bottom of your feet to your belly, then from your hands toward your shoulders, and finally, upward on your torso toward your heart to encourage lymphatic drainage, which collects near your heart.

☐ **Epsom salts.** Buy a large bag of Epsom salts and your favorite aromatherapy oils. A nightly bath truly helps highly sensitive people (myself included!) create a buffer from the day. Make a hot detox bath at least five times per week, and add one cup of Epsom salts (magnesium sulfate) plus ten to twenty drops of essential oil (my favorites are sandalwood, frankincense, and lavender). About 72 percent of women are deficient in magnesium (as measured in your red blood cells), which can prevent your DNA from methylating (an important and good action your body takes to support your genes) and increase the accumulation of bad estrogens. Research shows that women with higher magnesium levels are leaner and have lower waist-to-hip ratios.[10] Taking an Epsom salts bath will help with this process; you'll methylate better and get rid of bad estrogens.

☐ **Tongue scraper.** Scraping your tongue each morning is a great way to get rid of some of the toxins that accumulate there overnight. And it helps with bad breath!

## Food Items

### *Produce*

☐ *Your favorite veggies (ideally organic, locally grown, and in season).* For example, stock up on lettuce, spinach, arugula, kale, broccoli, Brussels sprouts, asparagus, beets, purple cabbage, cabbage, celery, and carrots. You will need a pound per day, so go ahead and weigh them in the store. You will need three pounds for the first three-day reset and a total of seven pounds each first week. I suggest that you keep three days' worth of vegetables in your refrigerator, make vegetable soup, and freeze the rest—just make sure your frozen vegetables don't contain sugar or additives.

☐ *Your favorite fruits (ideally organic, locally grown, and in season).* Keep lemons in stock, because you'll be drinking lemon water daily. Buy plenty of avocados, olives (whole and puréed as a tapenade), fresh and dried coconut, and berries. Limit high-glycemic fruits if you are trying to lose weight (I define low-glycemic fruits based on their fructose content, and these include avocados, olives, coconut, lemons, and berries), and eliminate high-glycemic fruits completely when you start the Fruitless reset (chapter 5).

### *Fridge and Freezer Items*

☐ *Organic and/or free-range chicken.*

☐ *Organic and/or free-range turkey.*

☐ *Organic and/or free-range eggs.*

☐ *Cold-water fish that are low in mercury.* Examples include wild Alaskan salmon, cod, snapper, tilapia, mackerel, trout, sardines, anchovies, orange roughy, herring, flounder, sturgeon, clams, crab, oysters, and scallops.

☐ *Hummus.*

### Pantry Items

☐ **Grain-free crackers, granola, etc.** Limit these if you are trying to lose weight. Some of my favorite brands include flackers from Doctor in the Kitchen (made from flax seeds) and raw, dehydrated vegetable crackers, such as those from Lydia's Organics (made from sprouted sunflower seeds, collards, carrots, celery, kale, spinach, zucchini, arugula, radicchio, and other natural ingredients).

☐ **Nuts and seeds.** For example, sunflower seeds, pumpkin seeds, raw almonds, cashews (limit if you're trying to lose weight because they are starchy), walnuts, and Brazil nuts.

☐ **Flax seeds, chia seeds, and/or hemp seeds.** These are excellent sources of additional fiber and nutrients.

☐ **Olive oil, avocado oil, coconut oil, and/or organic ghee.** Olive and avocado oils are best for low-temperature cooking or raw dressings. Coconut oil is suitable for high-temperature cooking and is also delicious in shakes! Ghee is clarified butter with the milk proteins removed. Avoid vegetable oils like canola, corn, and soy.

☐ **Coconut aminos.** These add a lot of flavor to steamed vegetables and soups. Find them online or at your local health food store.

☐ **Apple cider vinegar and red wine vinegar.**

☐ **Fresh and dried herbs and spices.** All herbs and spices are allowed, as long as they don't contain sugar or additives. Examples include tarragon, basil, thyme, parsley, cilantro, ginger, shiso leaf, cayenne, cinnamon, garlic, and onion.

☐ **Extra-dark chocolate.** Purchase 80 percent cacao or higher. Omit if it's an avalanche food that you can't stop eating.

### Beverages

☐ *Filtered water.* Use water for smoothies, and drink a large glass (8 to 12 ounces) with one tablespoon of apple cider vinegar and/or toss in pieces of fresh vegetables or fruit (lemon, lime, berries).

☐ *Sparkling water.* Sparkling water with fresh lemon, mint, or a small amount of frozen berries is a great alternative to soda or sugary juices.

☐ *Unsweetened almond, coconut, or hemp milk.* Use these milks for smoothies.

☐ *Hot water with lemon and cayenne.* You'll be drinking hot water with cayenne daily, first thing in the morning, during your Hormone Reset. It will alkalinize your body, and you may be surprised to find that this morning ritual is enough to replace your usual morning cup o' joe (or tea).

☐ *Hydrosols.* I love to drink hydrosols that combine small amounts of plant extract, at low concentrations, in sparkling water. I make my own by adding a few drops of essential oil, such as lavender, mint, or rose, to my water.

☐ *Coconut kefir.* Buy it online or make it yourself (see Resources). Coconut kefir is a nondairy combination of coconut water, a small amount of sugar (to feed the cultures), and a "starter" kit to inoculate with healthy bacteria.

☐ *Herbal teas.* Some of my favorites are ayurvedic teas. Choose from the large selection of herbal teas that help you with balancing your hormones or sleep. I love licorice tea. Aveda's Comforting Tea is my preferred iced tea. I brew it double strength and serve it over ice. Hands down, my favorite hot tea is organic chocolate herbal tea. Search online or go to your local health food store. I like Tisano and Republic of Tea brands.

# Dr. Sara's Reset Guidelines

## EAT/DRINK

- **Water:** Drink at least 2.2 liters per day for women (3 liters for men). Other approved beverages include hot water with lemon and herbal teas.

- **Vegetables:** Aim for one pound per day—half lightly cooked, half raw. (If you have thyroid problems you may wish to lightly cook all your vegetables.)

- **Clean proteins:** Eat 25 to 40 grams of protein per meal, aiming for 75 to 125 grams total per day, or about 25 to 33 percent of your total calories: Enjoy eating crustaceans, cold-water fish, organic and pastured chicken and eggs, and limited non-GM soy and legumes.

- **Net carbohydrates:** Eat 25 to 49 grams of net carbohydrates (total carbohydrates less fiber, in grams) per day. Include sweet potatoes, yams, cassava, lotus root, plantains, and Hormone Reset shakes. Overall, net carbohydrates should be 10 to 15 percent of total calories each day, which ends up including 10 to 25 percent of total calories from slow carbohydrates, as long as you're consuming sufficient fiber.

- **Healthy fats:** Eat the remaining calories in fat, or about one-half of your total calories. Consume seafood, avocados, and olives, and cook food in coconut oil and pastured ghee.

## MOVE

- Aim to get **at least 30 minutes per day** of movement or exercise.

- **Listen to your body:** If you feel like running, great! If you want to do something more low-key, honor that.

- Generally, lighter forms of exercise—such as **yoga or walking**—work best.

## SUPPLEMENT

**Fiber:** Work up slowly to 35 to 45 grams per day for women (40 to 50 grams for men). Don't increase more than 5 grams per day in order to prevent gas and bloating!

**Dr. Sara's Hormone Reset Kit** is available at www.HormoneReset.com/supplements and can help you detoxify more deeply.

**Shakes:** Buy a nondairy, nonwhey protein powder for making an optional one to two shakes per day, such as the shake I personally vetted in Dr. Sara's Hormone Reset Kit.

## Final Word

It's easy to rush into things, but rushing doesn't usually lead to changes that stick. It's a more advanced practice to take things slowly and tethered to your intention. That's what prep is all about. It's about honoring your choice to create your personal Hormone Reset and making sure that you are preparing yourself for success. Now that you know how the Hormone Reset works—what to measure, what to buy, what to eat and not eat, what to do and not do— you're prepared for the first reset. Remember, this is not a restrictive diet. We are going to address the root causes of why you can't lose weight by correcting your hormonal misfires. It's an innovative way to totally transform your body from the inside out. Let's fix your broken metabolism and burn fat so you can get lean and healthy again, starting with Meatless, the three-day reset for estrogen!

# PART TWO

# The Seven Hormonal Resets

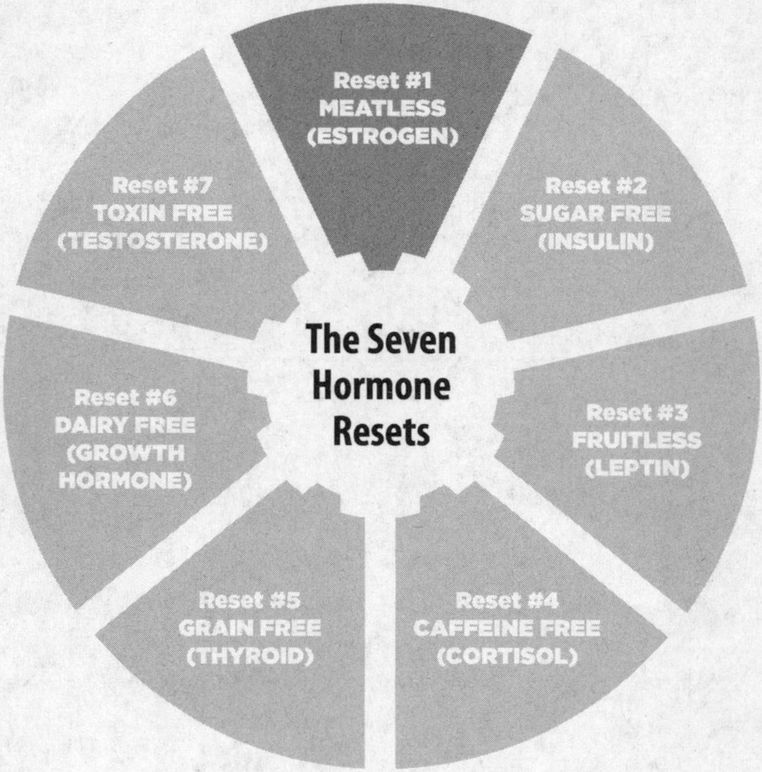

The Seven Hormone Resets

Reset #1
MEATLESS
(ESTROGEN)

Reset #2
SUGAR FREE
(INSULIN)

Reset #3
FRUITLESS
(LEPTIN)

Reset #4
CAFFEINE FREE
(CORTISOL)

Reset #5
GRAIN FREE
(THYROID)

Reset #6
DAIRY FREE
(GROWTH
HORMONE)

Reset #7
TOXIN FREE
(TESTOSTERONE)

# CHAPTER 3

# Meatless

ESTROGEN RESET: *Days 1 to 3*

My husband loves meat. He knows the ethical, environmental, and health arguments against it, but he adores red meat washed down with red wine. He's not alone: according to the U.S. Department of Agriculture, meat consumption is at an all-time high. In 2000, we ate 195 pounds per person, and that's 57 pounds more than in the 1950s.[1] Even though I think of meat eaters as being mainly men—I imagine cavemen circling a wild animal they just hunted and caught—it's fascinating to me how modern meat is the food that disturbs estrogen balance the most. Since women have far more estrogen than men, that means we're more vulnerable to the effects of meat (and alcohol), which raises estrogen. Even if you're not a meat eater, start with this reset so you can get your estrogen back into balance.

Estrogen is the hormone primarily responsible for making us uniquely women, with breasts, hips, curves, and glossy locks; that is, we're not simply small men. Yet there's something freaky that happens when you're female and you eat grain-fed, hormone-injected, superbug-infected meat: it slows down your digestion and may make you bloated or constipated (or both!); it raises your body's estrogen levels; and it messes with your microbiome, the collective DNA of the microbes that live in your gut and elsewhere in your body. Here is the biological principle: while it's true that meat has a higher fat content than other sources of protein, the bigger problem is *what's hidden in the fat of most meats* you find at your grocery store. You are anciently hardwired by your own DNA and microbiome to eat mostly vegetables, nuts, seeds, the occasional fruit, and clean proteins, regardless of your blood type and ethical views. In fact, such native and unprocessed foods keep you lean and your hormones in balance, particularly estrogen.

Unfortunately, rapid changes in industrial agriculture and cultural expectations over the past century have outpaced the ability of our genes to adapt. Consequently, obesity rates have nearly tripled in the United States since the 1960s.[2] Agricultural policies were changed in the 1970s, allowing our government to subsidize corn and soy—which is fed to cattle to accelerate the production of meat and dairy—to the tune today of $30 billion per year. Meat used to be a luxury to my great-grandmother, born in 1900. She would get it from the local butcher on Fridays, and it was fresh from a local ranch. Now we expect meat daily and consider it a sign of affluence. Today, 95 percent of food is grown and processed by industrial agriculture. Put simply, our DNA-driven biology hasn't yet adjusted to modern meat, and women are particularly at risk from the effect of meat on their estrogen.

In this chapter, you will review the specific role of estrogen and how it behaves and feels in your body when it's out of balance and accelerating the growth of your fat cells. You'll learn how to activate estrogen with food in a positive manner so it stops making you fat.

## Self-Assessment

Is your out-of-balance estrogen the reason for your inability to lose weight? Complete the following self-assessment to find out. Do you have or have you experienced in the past six months . . .

☐ Difficulty with weight loss? Rapid weight gain, particularly in the hips and butt?

☐ Bloating or fluid retention?

☐ Consumption of conventional meat? Do you eat at least one meal away from home per week?

☐ Treatments with oral hormones (birth control pills or hormone replacement medication—even bioidentical hormones) or antibiotics?

☐ Soreness when you (or a massage therapist or reflexologist) press in the hollow on top of your foot, between your big toe and second toe? (This is called the LV3 point, and in Chinese medicine, it becomes sensitive to pressure when you have liver stagnation, one of the symptoms of estrogen dominance.)

☐ Autoimmune conditions, in which your immune system attacks your own tissues, such as Hashimoto's disease (autoimmune thyroiditis)?

☐ Large or increased bra-cup size or breast tenderness?

☐ Abnormal Pap smears? Heavy bleeding or postmenopausal bleeding? Fibroids? Endometriosis or painful periods? (Endometriosis occurs when pieces of the uterine lining grow outside the uterine cavity, such as on the ovaries or bowel, and cause painful periods.)

☐ Mood swings, PMS, depression, or just irritability? Weepiness, sometimes over the most ridiculous things? Mini breakdowns? Anxiety?

☐ Frequent migraines or other headaches?

☐ A red flush or frequent blushing on your face (or a diagnosis of rosacea), triggered by heat, skin products, red wine, spicy foods, or dairy?

☐ Gallbladder problems (or removal)?

*Interpret Your Results*

- **If you have five or more of these symptoms,** you are very
  likely estrogen dominant (a state when you have too much
  estrogen compared with its counterhormone, progesterone).
  Estrogen is most likely keeping you from getting lean. I urge you
  to address this hormone imbalance by following the instructions
  in this chapter, since estrogen dominance puts you at significant
  risk for weight gain, breast cancer, prediabetes, and diabetes.
  Women at the greatest risk are between the ages of thirty-five
  and fifty, when the ovaries make less progesterone, allowing
  estrogen to dominate. (Men can develop estrogen dominance
  too, as they age, which leads to fatty deposits on the breasts,
  hips, and love handles.) I recommend asking your doctor for
  a test of your estrogen and progesterone levels (see the Test
  Yourself section, page 72).

- **If you have fewer than five of these symptoms or are
  unsure,** perform this reset, whether you're a meat eater or not,
  so we can determine if you are estrogen dominant.

When I completed my medical training, no one talked about
estrogen dominance. They weren't ignoring it; I simply don't think
anyone knew anything about it. I was taught to prescribe birth
control pills for women with ill-defined hormone problems up
until age fifty, and hormone replacement therapy after that. I
knew that birth control pills balanced out women who had too
much estrogen, so the term "estrogen dominance" had a context
in my mind. But as I learned more about the particular issues
women face—difficulty losing weight, breast tenderness, ovarian
cysts, premenstrual syndrome, endometrial polyps, fibroids,
endometriosis—I realized that estrogen dominance was the
elephant in the room that most of modern medicine was not
addressing, and meat consumption plays a key role. With this
chapter, my hope is to right this wrong.

# Estrogen Dominance Is Personal

Even though I'm a medical doctor, I didn't know I had estrogen dominance until my midthirties, when I couldn't lose the baby fat. To get back to my pre-pregnancy weight, I became increasingly desperate and decided to try eating only raw food for ninety days. Although I had more energy eating this way, I felt like a slave to the endless preparation it took to make my meals. Not to mention that it cramped my social life: I was the weird guest at the dinner party who couldn't eat anything the hostess offered and pulled out my own little glass containers of organic vegetables from my purse. To add insult to injury, I didn't even lose weight!

After three months of eating raw, I decided to change course and shifted to being a vegan—no animal products, not even eggs. I probably didn't get enough protein because my energy soon plummeted, and I felt even worse than when I had a newborn and was a sleepless zombie. It turned out that my iron was low, so I couldn't get oxygen to my brain or muscles. Although I didn't lose weight eating vegan, I did have some significant changes to my body: the fat from my breasts had mysteriously moved to my waist. Not exactly the change I had hoped might happen!

At the same time I was struggling with my resistance to weight loss, I noticed that many of my patients had similar challenges. They told me South Beach didn't work anymore. They were tired of Atkins and all that meat. Like me, they felt stuck. They would start a new diet on a Monday with great intentions, and by Wednesday, they went to bed lost, angry, and frustrated that they couldn't muster the willpower to restrict the calories or the carbs.

Since veganism wasn't working for me, I had the idea to start adding fish and crustaceans, and within a matter of days, I lost 5 pounds. I knew I was onto something, and I presumed seafood offered a better type of protein or fat for me. Then I added anti-inflammatory meat, like wild game (elk, moose, and wild bison), pastured eggs, bone broths, and grass-fed beef. My iron normalized, and I wasn't as tired. I stopped eating conventional meat at restaurants, which often cook foods in industrial seed oils—a deadly, inflammatory combination. Industrial seed oils are linked to higher rates of inflammation and problems with insulin and leptin—and they flip the hormone metabolic switch to make you fat.

I was making progress, but it wasn't until I passed on the alcohol for three weeks and started eating a pound of vegetables per day that my estrogen got back to its rightful place. I lost 25 pounds and became lean and energized.

I've been where you might be: hopeless and perhaps somewhat despondent about looking plump and middle-aged well before your time. By taking control of your meat and alcohol consumption in the first three-day reset, you can have similar results. In this chapter, we'll focus on how going meatless jump-starts a series of beneficial events in your body that triggers your estrogen system to reboot. If you're like the majority of overweight women that I've counseled with excess estrogen, the weight falls away. Addressing your estrogen overload by abstaining from eating meat is the first step toward fixing your broken metabolism.

## The Science Behind Meatless

The connection between meat and estrogen is profound. When you eat conventionally raised red meat, estrogen overload is more likely. When you go meatless, your estrogen decreases. Not surprisingly, vegetarians have the edge here. That could be due to the hormones in the meat, the type of bacteria cultivated in the guts of people who eat a lot of meat,[3] or a combination of factors. We do know that a meat-based diet is linked to higher body mass index and that too much of the wrong type of saturated fat raises estrogen.

Fiber is shown to help you lose weight, feel full, and stabilize your blood sugar, yet meat eaters consume half as much fiber as vegetarians.[4] On average, omnivores eat 12 grams of fiber each day, and vegetarians consume 26 grams per day. Vegetarians poop more volume and excrete three times the amount of estrogen as meat eaters, thereby preventing estrogen overload. In fact, estrogen levels in the blood of vegetarians are 15 to 20 percent lower than those of omnivores.[5]

Higher estrogen in women arises from greater lifetime estrogen exposure and recirculation in the gut and blood, like bad karma. I'm here as your coach to flip your "switch" on estrogen, which allows you to reduce the estrogen pollution in your body and hopefully prevent the risk of estrogen-dominant conditions such as diabetes, metabolic syndrome, and certain forms of breast, ovarian, and endometrial cancer. Scientists know that estrogen dominance is a common root cause of these conditions, especially when a woman menstruates early, becomes obese, has never borne a child, or enters menopause at a later age. The reasons to go meatless are evident. When you reverse your estrogen dominance, you clear the path toward a healthy weight.

## Track Your Burger

If you're not yet convinced of the connection between modern meat and excess estrogen, come with me on a quick trip through your digestion of a freshly grilled hamburger from your neighbor's barbecue so you may grasp how meat disrupts your body.

As you smell the aroma of the burgers cooking on the grill, you may be unaware that they were previously part of cows raised in concentrated animal feeding operations (CAFOs) and fed grain, typically genetically modified corn rather than grass, and highly stressed.

Your neighbor asks if you want the burger on a bun. You decline (and pat yourself on the back because you like to wrap your burger in lettuce and save the carbs). As a plate is passed to you with the burger and a single leaf of lettuce, you add ketchup and a little pickle relish. You eye the burger with anticipation, and you don't think about how the standard practice for cattle is to treat them prophylactically with antibiotics and dewormers, thereby breeding bacterial and parasite resistance and leading to the rise of superbugs, which can trigger hard-to-treat infections and foodborne illnesses. The practice began with poultry in the 1940s, when farmers found that antibiotics fattened chickens. In the United States, 70 percent of antibiotics are currently used for livestock, mostly for "growth promotion." Rates of superbug contamination are alarming: the Environmental Working Group determined that 55 percent of beef, 69 percent of pork, and 81 percent of turkey meat contains superbugs.[6]

Your first bite of the burger may taste juicy and satisfying, but it's a false satiety because lurking in the meat are several problems, including the following:

- *Steroid hormones.* On average, six steroid hormones are pumped into feedlot cattle in order to fatten them up so there's more income per animal. As you chew the burger, you're consuming the same growth hormones, and they'll fatten you up too.

- *Persistent organic pollutants (POPs).* These are synthetic chemicals that may act as xenoestrogens (or fake estrogens) in the body and raise your level of endogenous estrogen, resulting in estrogen dominance. Examples are polychlorinated biphenyls (PCBs) and dioxins.[7] Additionally, several have been shown to open up the gut barrier—causing leaky gut and inflammation, and shifting the microbiome in the wrong direction—and may contribute to breast cancer.

- *Poor nutrient density.* Grain-fed meat is lower in vitamins A, B, C, and E; conjugated linoleic acid (found to hasten fat burning); and beneficial omega-3s; plus it's higher in omega-6 fatty acids compared with meat from pastured or wild animals. In comparisons of omega-3 levels in grass-fed versus grain-fed

meat, *grass-fed meat contained up to ten times more omega-3.*
What's important is your overall ratio of omega-6 to omega-3; that is, too much omega-6 compared with omega-3 leads to inflammation and more fat storage. Grain-fed beef shows a ratio of eight to one, whereas grass-fed beef averages two to one. (CAFO-raised chicken is even more problematic with a ratio of nineteen to one, whereas pastured chicken has a ratio of approximately eleven to one.)[8]

- *Genetically modified grains.* Often GM corn is used to feed animals, and consuming those animals may also cause leaky gut and hormone disruption.

As if that list weren't scary enough, when you eat fat from conventional animal meat, these toxins enter your gut and are sent to the liver. Your liver doesn't know what to do with them, so they're sent to the fat stores, accumulating and magnifying in quantity over time. It's like the dresser in your spare bedroom: you put things in the drawers that you don't need. Your body does this to protect your organs from toxic overload, but the strategy backfires when you accumulate too much. Just as the dresser drawers may overflow and become hard to close, your fat tissue eventually starts to release more toxins into your bloodstream, which is tied to obesity, insulin resistance, and breast cancer. As your tissue releases toxins, your body gets the message to store even more fat—and because fat cells produce estrogen, your estrogen burden climbs higher still. Ultimately, estrogen dominance causes overweight women to store more fat instead of burning it and changes the microbiome to pull more energy out of food for storage, not fuel.

Back to that ketchup and lone lettuce leaf on your plate: most people who consume a typical Western diet high in meat don't eat enough vegetables (ketchup doesn't count!), which are rich in fiber and micronutrients—and both counter the estrogen pollution of dirty meat and protect you from bioaccumulation and biomagnification. In other words, too much conventional meat and too little fiber from vegetables combine as a double whammy that makes you fat, toxic, and resistant to weight loss. Instead of one lettuce leaf, you need to consume one pound of vegetables each day.

Halfway through the burger, you pause to praise your neighbor on the yummy barbecue, and he offers you a glass of chardonnay or a mojito. Sadly, alcohol makes the whole excess estrogen problem worse. Oblivious, you toast your neighbor and wash down your next bite of burger. You tell yourself, "Okay, just one glass, since I had two glasses every night this past week." Boom! You just upped your risk of breast cancer.

Look, if you love meat and/or alcohol, I get it. Frankly, my mouth is watering as I write about grilled burgers. The good news is that by removing meat and alcohol for the next three days, and then continuing for the full twenty-one day program, you can finally lose that stubborn weight. This will initiate a virtuous chain reaction—starting first with estrogen but then later involving other hormones, such as insulin (detailed in chapter 4) and leptin (detailed in chapter 5). It's time to push the reset button on estrogen—clear out meat, toxins and contaminants, and alcohol—and finally begin to get lean.

## Estrogen and Progesterone: Fire and Ice

We've established that estrogen is what makes you feminine. When it's in the normal zone relative to its counterpart—progesterone— estrogen makes you feel happy, sane, slim, and emotionally connected. These hormones are like fire and ice, and when in balance, progesterone is the ice that keeps the fire of estrogen under control.

My research and experience reveal that the majority of women who struggle with their weight have estrogen dominance, especially after age thirty-five, when progesterone begins to wane. Red meat and alcohol exacerbate the imbalance. Pursuing our analogy further, there's too much fire and not enough ice. You make too much estrogen, and not enough progesterone. The increased fire is not a good thing: it creates inflammation in the body that can be hidden but causes fat loss resistance, mood problems, and gut issues.

Estrogen dominance isn't just a problem of increased estrogen levels in your body. It can also result from high or low levels of other hormones like excess insulin, medical problems like obesity (fat cells make estrogen), and other environmental exposures, such as skin care products and plastics. We will address these concerns in future chapters.

## How Insulin and Estrogen Can Block Metabolism

One reason that estrogen dominance is connected to fat-loss resistance is because of the cross talk between two important hormones of metabolism: insulin and estrogen. When you are insulin resistant, which means your cells can't absorb the extra blood glucose your body keeps generating from the food you eat, your liver converts the glucose into fat (see chapter 4, page 86). Those extra fat cells are now extraneous estrogen-making laboratories. Rather than being your best friend, excess estrogen does a backflip and wreaks havoc on your ability to burn and lose fat. The best pattern interrupt is to eliminate meat (and alcohol) and increase fiber.

To make matters worse, beginning in your early forties you become resistant to estrogen because your receptors go into semi-retirement and your estrogen levels climb higher to try to get the attention of those receptors. As a result, your memory falters, you feel irritable, and fat attaches like Krazy Glue to your waist. You are now officially resistant to fat loss, regardless of your weight, and it gets even worse in menopause.

Put it all together, and you can understand why so many women begin to experience slow metabolism and fat-loss resistance after age forty. The solution is to forgo meat and alcohol and consume one pound of vegetables per day.

The bottom line: too much estrogen keeps you fat by creating a vicious cycle, which must be broken to help you lose weight permanently.

### ESTROGEN DOMINANCE AND MENOPAUSE

*When I broach the topic of estrogen dominance with postmenopausal women, they bristle and tell me they are past all of that. They think of estrogen as a young woman's hormone, responsible only for menstruation, mood swings, and fertility. Nothing could be further from the truth. Regardless of your age, it's crucial to understand estrogen and how it is working in your body. Too much estrogen relative to progesterone can cause mood problems, bloating, fibroids, insomnia, and anxiety at any age—until you die. In addition (I'll repeat myself so that it sinks in),* **estrogen dominance is the main reason women have a harder time losing weight regardless of age when compared with men. Lest you are still fuzzy, too much estrogen causes weight gain.**

*Estrogen, along with other hormones, is responsible for how you respond to food, drink, and supplements. The seven metabolic hormones determine whether the food you eat is burned or stored as fat. So, instead of dismissing this hormone, I implore you to understand what it does and its central role in your weight loss.*

---

## The Vicious Cycle of Estrogen Dominance

When you understand that being overweight involves more than just how much you eat and how little you exercise, you have an advantage in the quest for a healthy body weight and lean body mass. That's because you've learned how to work with the innate intelligence of your body instead of against it. I've found that when estrogen dominance is the primary reason for weight gain and weight retention, most of those women eat large amounts of conventional red meat and cheese, crave refined carbohydrates such as french fries (and don't get the fiber they need to guide estrogen expertly through the body), juggle tons of stress, and drink too much alcohol. The result is that estrogen dominance blocks their metabolism—the speed with which they burn calories—in several ways.

First, their microbiome has too many fat bugs (bacteria that hang onto fat) and not enough skinny bugs (bacteria that promote the burning of fat). Second, omnivorous women with estrogen excess don't remove that excess in their bowel movements like women who eat a more plant-based diet—which contains more fiber and stimulates removal of excess estrogen. Third, estrogen dominance makes a woman more likely to have bloating and constipation. Finally, women who eat red meat have higher rates of blood sugar problems, as indicated in a recent large-scale study of red meat consumption, diabetes, and metabolic syndrome in nearly a hundred and fifty thousand people, published in the prestigious *Journal of the American Medical Association*.[9] However, this study was observational and didn't prove that red meat is the cause of blood sugar problems.

Other studies suggest that processed meat may be the greater evil.[10] Research shows that processed meats (meats that have gone through a chemical process to extend shelf life, including ham, hot dogs, lunch meats, sausage, and ham hocks) are full of nitrates and nitrites, and are associated with diabetes, accelerated cellular aging, and cancer.[11] Indeed, one study showed that ham worsens blood sugar far more than eggs.[12]

If you wonder why it's so hard for you to lose weight when a friend or spouse sees pounds melt away on the exact same eating plan, it's likely you have different root causes of fatness. Over the next seventy-two hours, as you start the Meatless reset, observe closely how much weight you lose. If you drop a significant amount—in the range of 3 to 5 pounds over three days of the first reset—bingo! You've found your first answer: your estrogen imbalance, caused by meat and alcohol, is keeping you fat.

If you are a woman with estrogen dominance, resetting your estrogen is a crucial piece of the puzzle. Fortunately, you hold the keys to the kingdom and can impact your estrogen ratio at any age. When you balance your estrogen and reset your ratio, you'll find a whole new relationship to food, weight, and your body.

## Paleo for Women Is Different than Paleo for Men

The Paleo diet has become very popular and emphasizes the consumption of vegetables, seeds, nuts, fruits, and meat like our Paleolithic ancestors ate. It also advocates avoiding the foods that came into our food chain later, such as grains, dairy, and legumes. It's true that our Paleolithic ancestors ate wild meat when they could find and catch it, and that it was anti-inflammatory. As discussed previously, today's meat offered at most grocery stores and restaurants is nothing like the wild game our ancestors ate—it *promotes inflammation* and makes us hoard fat. Because we women are so efficient at fat storage, I believe that's a common reason why Paleo doesn't give women the results that men enjoy when it comes to losing weight, getting lean, and reducing inflammation.

In short, conventional meat isn't a woman's best choice. To find out if meat is making you fat, give it up for three days and let your body (and the bathroom scale) inform your relationship to meat.

On the other hand, I don't believe that a one-size-fits-all is the right approach for women to get lean. As you perform the Meatless reset, keep in mind that many women find that their energy lags when they cut out meat. The key, once again, is to cultivate body awareness and to use this reset to discover your response to meat and alcohol. Former President Bill Clinton found that when he began following a vegan food plan after his heart attack he was too tired and couldn't keep up with his grueling schedule. He added salmon and eggs, and that boosted his energy. Clean proteins like pastured eggs and wild-caught fish are excellent choices when you're resetting your estrogen load.

## Disrupt Your Estrogen

As you've learned, hormones are the master switches of metabolism, and they tell your cells what to do. Therefore, the key to keeping your metabolism humming is not to do the same old thing day after day but to disrupt the status quo. When it comes to resetting your estrogen levels, you need to do so sporadically. You want to shuffle your body's organizational chart so that your estrogen works more efficiently than before.

Receptors take seventy-two hours to turn over. In the next three days, you'll start by removing red meat from your diet and replacing it with clean vegetables, fiber, and proteins that help balance your estrogen. You'll stay off of meat and alcohol for the full twenty-one days. Without meat weighing you down, you'll fill up on veggies and filtered water, priming your system for resetting your estrogen for good. You'll change the bacteria in your gut that might be contributing to estrogen dominance by encouraging more *Prevotella* compared with the *Firmicutes* phylum of bacteria,[13] a favorable shift that may be linked to weight loss.[14]

Since you're on a fast track to weight loss, I want you to support these changes by getting rid of other causes of estrogen dominance: dump the alcohol on Day 1, and begin to wean off caffeine. (Caffeine is linked to estrogen dominance, and removing it causes withdrawal symptoms, so I urge you to begin the slow wean now in order to be off caffeine by Day 10, the cortisol reset.)

By going meatless, you're not only addressing your weight by resetting the hormones of metabolism, you're also potentially saving your life. I'm not being dramatic here. Too much estrogen gives you a greater risk of breast cancer. Ask cancer researchers what they eat. Usually the answer is vegetables; no meat; no sugar; plant sources of fat, such as olive and coconut oil; and healthy proteins, such as nuts, seeds (like quinoa), and wild-caught salmon.

I'm not claiming that all meat is bad, but there are powerful arguments to limit your consumption of conventional meat. Beyond the link to a greater risk of diabetes, breast cancer, and metabolic syndrome, there's the harm to the environment. Raising livestock requires high water usage (at the time of writing, California is experiencing a severe drought) and contributes significantly to increased greenhouse gases because of the massive release of methane gas from cattle (i.e., cow farts). In fact, a pound of red meat requires 2,500 gallons of water versus 23 gallons to produce a pound of lettuce.

Try substituting other protein sources, such as fish, crustaceans, pastured eggs, pastured chicken, and lentils, because they will help you reset estrogen and your microbiome.

There's no such thing as humanely produced meat. There's more humane and less humane, but keep in mind that currently in the United States, 9.8 billion animals are raised annually for food and slaughtered.[15] Allow me to do the math: that's 26.8 million animals slaughtered per day, and 1 million per hour. Our passion for meat is relentless, unhealthy, and inhumane. Over the next three days, connect with your compassion for animals.

# Meatless: The Three-Day Reset for Estrogen

The goal of this chapter is to reset your estrogen by having you forgo meat and alcohol plus boost your fiber intake for three days in order to promote fat loss. The directions are simple: skip eating meat for three days, eat a pound of vegetables daily, and increase your fiber intake by 5 grams per day. These small steps will yield dramatic results.

## MEATLESS RULES: DO THESE EACH DAY

1. **Forgo meat and alcohol.** Eat a minimum of one pound of vegetables per day, divided over three meals, with healthy proteins. One pound of vegetables is approximately five to ten cups, depending on the vegetables, whether raw or cooked (I recommend a 50/50 split). Not sure how to fit in so many vegetables? Make vegetable soup. Find some of my favorite recipes that are delicious plus chock-full of fresh vegetables and fiber in the Recipes section (page 267).

   *Food List:* Lentils, beans of all types, nuts, nut butters (such as almond butter and cashew butter), seeds, cold-water fish that are low in mercury (cod, salmon, tilapia, mackerel, sardines), shellfish, and pastured chicken and eggs. For nutrient-dense vegetables, choose greens like kale, Swiss chard, collards, watercress, bok choy, cabbage, spinach, arugula, and chicory. Other vegetables include broccoli, radish, turnip, carrots, squash, bell pepper, kohlrabi, and cauliflower.

2. **Increase your fiber intake by 5 grams per day,** to an optimal range of 35 to 45 grams per day (40 to 50 grams per day for men). Increased dietary fiber improves the ability of the liver to clear excess estrogen—that is, more fiber lowers estrogen levels in the body—and you poop more estrogen out of your system. For example, with one cup of steamed broccoli and one cup of lentils for lunch, you'll get 22 grams of fiber. While you might be enticed

by the plethora of "fiber-rich" packaged foods such as breads and cereals found throughout your grocery store, please stick to fiber that grows naturally. It turns out that along with added fiber, most of these processed foods have added sugar and salt too.

*Food List:* Soaked chia seeds, freshly ground flax seeds, organic vegetables (especially spinach, kale, and other greens), lentils, legumes, low-glycemic fruit (berries), and fiber capsules and powders (to be added to shakes).

3. **Eat good fats.** When you give up toxic meat, you have the opportunity to fill up on healthy fats instead. When I began learning about nutrition in the 1980s, there was a prevailing myth that eating fat makes you fat and clogs your arteries. The truth is that there's good and bad fat, but it doesn't break down along the lines that you might think. Saturated fat is not the villain. There are good and bad types of saturated fat, just as there are good and bad types of polyunsaturated fatty acids (PUFAs). Keep this rule in mind: eat natural, unprocessed fat that's present in whole foods. Healthy saturated fats include organic coconut oil and virgin red palm oil (not to be confused with red palm kernel oil), which are the best oils for cooking because they are stable at higher temperatures, plus they taste delicious! PUFAs from whole foods make the membranes of your cells more flexible and heal your metabolism. Avoid damaged, industrial PUFAs such as corn, cottonseed, safflower, and soybean oils. For some people, like myself, a variation in the PPARG gene provides weight loss benefits when you consume more of the good PUFAs compared with saturated fat. In other words, I lose weight when I eat fish instead of burgers.

*Food List:* Healthy sources of polyunsaturated fats include cold water fish (salmon, halibut, mackerel), crustaceans (oysters, shrimp, crab), borage and evening primrose oil, pastured ghee (clarified butter), nuts and nut oils (pine nuts, walnuts, almonds), poultry and pastured eggs, and seeds (chia, flax, sunflower). Healthy sources of monounsaturated fats include avocados, dark chocolate (80 percent or more cacao), duck fat, nuts and nut butters (macadamias, cashews, pistachios, pecans), olive oil, avocado oil, macadamia oil, olives, seeds (pumpkin, sesame). Healthy saturated fats come from coconut oil, medium chain triglyceride (MCT) oil, and red palm oil.

### SAMPLE MENU

Here is a suggested menu for resetting your estrogen. For nutritional data, check out the Notes section.[16]

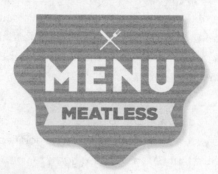

**BREAKFAST**

1 cup lightly brewed green or white tea (begin to wean off caffeine)

Omelet made with 3 eggs, ½ cup asparagus, and 1 cup chopped spinach cooked in 1 tablespoon coconut oil

**LUNCH**

Detox Shake made with 1 cup unsweetened almond milk, 1 cup chopped kale, 1 tablespoon MCT oil (see Recipes)

1 cup chopped bell peppers

1 ounce raw cashews (approximately 15 to 20)

Cashew nuts

**DINNER**

6 ounces wild-caught salmon (slightly bigger than the size of your fist)

1 cup lightly steamed broccoli

2 cups salad with 2 tablespoons oil and red wine vinegar to taste (example: 1 cup chopped artichoke hearts, ½ cup chopped purple cabbage, and ½ cup torn romaine lettuce)

## SOY: RULES OF ENGAGEMENT

*Soy has been popular for more than five thousand years in Asia. Why have we recently demonized it and made the choice to consume soy endlessly confusing? Sometimes I will order tempeh while out to dinner with friends, and they stare at me in horror, convinced that I will become estrogen dominant and develop breast cancer overnight, and that my thyroid will stop working. I disagree: small amounts of whole soy, preferably organic and fermented, have been shown to be a great choice when you go meatless. Allow me to unravel the mysteries of soy and offer sane, evidence-based rules of engagement.*

*Here are my recommendations:*

*__Avoid GM soy.__ Genetically modified (GM) soy crops were widely introduced in 1996, and today up to 94 percent of soy available in American grocery stores has been genetically modified. Unfortunately, there is evidence that GM crops cause harm to your gut, microbiome, sex hormones (including aromatase, which is involved in estrogen synthesis), and insulin. For this reason, I assume GM soy is guilty of harm to your body until proven innocent, and I advise you to avoid it by choosing organic whole soy or soy that is labeled "Non-GMO."*

*__Eat whole soy.__ In Asian countries, people eat moderate amounts of whole soy as part of a healthy diet. In the United States, Big Food pushes weird and highly processed foods under the guise that it's healthy. Does "soy protein isolate" sound like a good idea? Instead of eating the whole-food version of soy, we try to isolate the "healthy" part, and it may be the reason behind the conflicting results, and by extension, the confusion about whether soy is good or bad for you.[17] I recommend eating only whole soy—not the isolates, not the processed version, but fresh soy food, such as organic tofu and edamame.*

*__Eat fermented soy,__ such as miso and tempeh. Several recent studies show that fermented soy at a dose of approximately 60 grams per day raises progesterone, lowers cholesterol, and prevents hyperglycemia.[18] Fermentation removes genetically modified components.*

*Short version: Don't let soy confuse you. Eat whole and non-GM soy, preferably fermented. If your thyroid is slow, limit yourself to two servings of whole soy per week.*

---

### From Dr. Sara's Case Files: Kristy, Age Forty

- *Lost 17 pounds in her Hormone Reset and 7 inches off her waist.*
- *In her version of the Hormone Reset, "wild-caught salmon replaced chicken nuggets. Fresh spinach replaced chocolate chip cookies."*
- *The first few days were rough. But soon something beautiful happened. She had energy—true energy. Not the shaky, temporary energy of coffee or sugar, but a real intrinsic fuel.*
- *Kristy started to notice other changes, such as no back pain or constipation. The weight began to fall off. Now she still doesn't eat sugar, rarely consumes alcohol and dairy, and she sleeps deeply and restfully.*
- *After completing her Hormone Reset, she lost another 28 pounds, for a total of 45 pounds lost.*

---

### WAYS TO WEAN YOURSELF OFF ALCOHOL

*When I completed my residency in obstetrics and gynecology in 1998 I was thirty-one and worked at a health maintenance organization (HMO). I was a bit of a purist and thrilled to practice the evidence-based medicine that I'd spent nine long years learning, night and day. I was assigned to a retiring physician and took over his practice of three thousand patients. It stunned me to find that most of them came in for their annual visits requesting Valium and other tranquilizers, so they could sleep and generally cope with a stressful life as a modern woman, and asking for a water pill, so they could deal with their fluid retention.*

I was shocked and more than a little judgmental. This wasn't the evidence-based medicine I had learned at Harvard Medical School and the University of California at San Francisco, where I'd served my residency. I didn't get it. What was everyone so strung out about? Then I turned thirty-five, and I completely got it.

When women are between the ages of thirty-five and fifty, many lose their sanity. I certainly did. As soon as I found myself in my mid thirties with two young kids, I finally understood the "It's the end of the day; I desperately need a drink to unwind" thing. You grab whatever you can to deal with the slowing metabolism and the growing difficulty coping with your life as you know it—full of bills, screaming children, demanding bosses, and spouses who feel equally spent. A glass of wine seems like just what the doctor ordered.

Not this doctor. I have faith that you can find ways to cope with the mounting stress without resorting to methods that halt your metabolism, use up your goodwill, and raise your bad estrogens. You can do this.

Carl Jung, M.D., the famous psychiatrist, said that a "craving for alcohol was the equivalent, on a low level, of the spiritual thirst of our being for wholeness, expressed in medieval language: the union with God." He continues: " . . . 'alcohol' in Latin is 'spiritus' and you use the same word for the highest religious experience as well as for the most depraving poison." I agree.

So, let's create wholeness and union with a Higher Power. Start by replacing "I must have a glass of _____ [fill in the blank]" with an alternative, such as "I'm going to try a different strategy that doesn't pump me full of bad, nasty estrogens." I love the idea my yoga teacher told me about samskaras, our conditioned patterns that create a groove in our minds. The more you repeat your habituated ways of thinking, the deeper the groove. Samskaras can be good or bad; it just depends on what you repeat. So, when you replace the negative thoughts with positive ones, you are making a new groove. In case you think this is some New Age baloney, I turn to the science of neuroplasticity, which basically says the same thing: the neurons that fire together, wire together.

My personal favorite exercise is to "take in the good," which I learned from neuropsychologist Dr. Rick Hanson, author of **Hardwiring Happiness.**[19]

1. **Have a positive experience.** This activates a positive mental state. Choose a positive experience that happened recently and consider it fully. Perhaps it was a physical pleasure, like inhaling roses on a walk, or an emotional pleasure, like feeling close to someone who matters to you.

2. **Enrich it.** Next, install the positive experience in your mind. Get a feeling for how it affected you on a sensory level—associated feelings of wellness, sights, smells, and how it made you feel. Allow yourself to open to the feeling and let it fill your body, mind, and spirit. As Dr. Hanson recommends, find something fresh or novel in it. Recognize how it could nourish you, which rewires your brain away from alcohol and toward what is good for you.

3. **Absorb it.** Let the positive feelings from this experience seep into you, providing soothing and calmness, filling you with gratitude and positive emotions. Create the intention that this feeling of being on your own side is sinking into you. Let the good become part of you. Surrender to it—not in a passive manner but in a way that serves your highest good.

This is self-directed neuroplasticity. You are rewiring your brain for pleasure that is not linked to alcohol. Make it a habit by practicing it daily for seventy-two hours.

---

## Supplements

Along with banishing alcohol and conventional meat, you can help to balance your estrogen levels with supplements, such as vitamin

B12, folate, magnesium, and an amino acid called methionine. These supplements can help produce good estrogens and decrease formation of bad estrogens. But if I had to pick only one supplement to get your estrogen back into balance, it's fiber: as I mentioned, women should consume 35 to 45 grams per day or more, and it is difficult to achieve those numbers with food alone.

For those of you suffering with hot flashes and night sweats as a result of estrogen imbalance, add Siberian rhubarb to your protocol. It's been shown in randomized trials—the best-quality evidence—to make women in perimenopause and menopause more comfortable, and it has an excellent safety profile.[20]

## Cell to Soul Practice

We compartmentalize as a survival instinct. We put health in one compartment, weight in another, relationship in a third compartment, and work in yet another. When it comes to our metabolic hormones, we can't afford to think of them separately. My hope is that you can integrate how you eat, move, think, and supplement so you can feel whole and alive, and feel that you are reaching your full potential.

My goal for you is to craft the best possible health. If you've been struggling with weight, body image, or erratic eating your whole life, I ask you to be gentle and to start with loving and kind words toward yourself. Even if it feels hokey, try it. As I hope you've learned by now, many of your health issues don't stem from the fact that you are weak or lazy or have no willpower. Your body might just need recalibration. So, stop blaming yourself, and put your energy into the positive direction of your own growth and healing.

*The Power of Positive Thinking* guru Norman Vincent Peale suggested that you list all your weaknesses, your failures, your doubts—everything negative—on a single piece of paper. On a second page, list all the good qualities you would like to have. Put away the first piece of paper and keep the second handy in your pocket or purse so you can read it over and over. Make an effort to edit and customize the statements I've included in the following meditation so that they work for you. Some people consider them a prayer for wholeness or a way to connect with a Higher Power.

## Your Homework: Loving-Kindness Meditation

This practice uses intention, words, imagery, and feelings to evoke loving-kindness toward yourself and others. When you repeat the script, you express an intention, planting the seeds of loving wishes.

To practice your loving-kindness meditation, sit comfortably and without distraction. Take five deep breaths with slow, long, and full exhalations.

State to yourself as a mantra the following:

*May I be filled with loving-kindness.*
*May I be happy.*
*May I be full of grace.*
*May I be healthy.*
*May I live with ease.*

Repeat as many times as you need to in order to feel complete. When you are ready, bring to mind a benefactor, someone it is easy to feel loving-kindness toward—perhaps a child or a pet—someone with whom you have an easy relationship. Have a sense of that being in your heart. Then begin to send blessings to the loved one:

*May you be filled with loving-kindness.*
*May you be happy.*
*May you be full of grace.*
*May you be healthy.*
*May you live with ease.*

Next, recite again for yourself:

*May I be filled with loving-kindness.*
*May I be happy.*
*May I be full of grace.*
*May I be healthy.*
*May I live with ease.*

For folks who've been practicing loving-kindness, it doesn't feel complete unless you extend the blessing to someone you've had a conflict with. Add a final phase of the meditation to someone you hold anger or resentment toward:

*May you be filled with loving-kindness.*
*May you be happy.*
*May you be full of grace.*
*May you be healthy.*
*May you live with ease.*

## Exercise

I have great news for those of you who hate to exercise! During the Meatless reset, I want to kick-start your metabolism with a simple goal: *sit less.* Rather than sweating for additional hours at the gym, begin to reset estrogen (and insulin) by sitting 90 minutes less each day. Several recent studies confirm the wisdom of reducing sedentary time—and even suggest it might be better than a vigorous workout.[21] These studies looked at patients with insulin resistance and found that the people with the least amount of time spent sitting, including time sitting at your desk or watching television, had lower blood sugar and cholesterol levels in addition to other risk factors for cardiovascular disease and diabetes. The benefit to health persisted for those who sat 90 minutes less than the control group, even after adjusting for time spent exercising.

While these studies do not prove a cause and effect between sitting less and reversal of estrogen dominance and insulin resistance, they suggest that we may need to redesign the current recommendations of 150 minutes of vigorous exercise per week for people with diabetes and ideally one hour per day (according to the Institute of Medicine of the National Academies and the International Association for the Study of Obesity). Vigorous exercise does help your mood, energy, brain, and focus, but it plays only a minor role in weight loss because it boosts appetite.

Here's how I sit less:

I write a lot, and for now, that means I'm mostly sitting. But before I sit, I do a set of twenty-five push-ups or twenty-five jumping jacks.

When I talk on the phone, I never sit. I walk around and climb the stairs in my home or office. It brings a whole new understanding to "phone it in."

Increasingly, I work at a stand-up desk. (My husband built one for me for less than $30, called an Ikea hack.)

When I sit, I work in sprint–recovery cycles. I set a timer on my smartphone that rings after fifty minutes, and I get up and move for ten minutes. Sometimes I sprint a few blocks near my home or perform a wall sit or do a few abdominal crunches.

Drink lots of filtered water—60 or more ounces per day—which will make you get up to pee once an hour.

Consider getting a treadmill desk! Many of my lean friends have one, and the idea is that you walk slowly while working at a standing desk. My brother-in-law just explained to me how to build one on the cheap, and it's easier than you might think.

Swing a kettlebell! I learned this one from Tim Ferriss, author of the *New York Times* bestseller *The 4-Hour Body*. Make sure you have good form by learning from an expert how to swing these heavy devices (mine weighs 35 pounds) so you don't injure yourself.

## Test Yourself

Based on your response to the self-assessment at the beginning of the chapter, you can start your estrogen reset without getting any laboratory testing beforehand. Your Meatless reset should improve your estrogen levels within seventy-two hours, but I'd like you to stay meatless (and alcohol free) for the full twenty-one days of the program. If you are not making the progress you had hoped for, consider talking to your practitioner about additional testing, such as your progesterone-to-estradiol ratio. Ask your clinician to measure your estradiol, the main estrogen, and your progesterone levels in your blood or saliva. You don't need a doctor's prescription in most locations.

## Notes from Hormone Resetters

"I'm utterly amazed at the person staring back at me in the mirror. I have lost weight and inches, but more amazingly, I feel so good. My skin is clear, my mood is steadier, my clothes are looser, and I feel energized to exercise. Now that I've gotten rid of my cravings, I feel like I can accomplish even more! I see each meal as an opportunity to nourish my body and not as an emotional experience to smooth the edges of a stressful day. Weekly (daily!) indulgences of dessert and wine don't appeal to me. I feel so empowered to make choices that make me feel good each and every day! Although I still feel I have too many stressors in my life, I feel totally equipped to handle them, and if my 'to do' list isn't finished, I am not defeated." —*Linda*

"For the first time in thirty years, I have started to lose weight. Previous to the first [Hormone Reset], I would sit at a level of going up and down in a 5-pound range. Now I am losing weight each week. I lost 12 pounds during the first [round] and 6 pounds this [round]. I did not put any weight back on after [my first time], and I am sure I will continue to lose pounds because I now have much better eating habits and understanding [of] what foods the body needs to be healthy. To me, as a breast cancer survivor, I feel like I have the world by the tail and that I have a great many happy and healthy years ahead." —*Judith*

"I'm pretty darn proud of having gone off the sugar and caffeine early and sticking with it! (Not to mention my pride in staying on the wagon since Day 1!) I am going to take the money I save from buying cocktails and buy myself something pretty when I hit my goal." —*Jeanine*

## Final Word

Recent research shows that an important way to reverse estrogen dominance in women is to connect with others. Closeness with a husband, partner, or girlfriend has been shown to raise progesterone levels in women, which ameliorates estrogen dominance. This makes sense to me, because I know that one of the best ways for stressed women to shift to a more proactive, energized, and buoyant mind-set is to connect with others, particularly women. This discovery explains why women "tend and befriend" as an effective way to cope with stress.

Care for yourself by making sure you take time out of your busy schedule to connect with your family and friends. This kind of attention will pay dividends to your well-being. You are worth it.

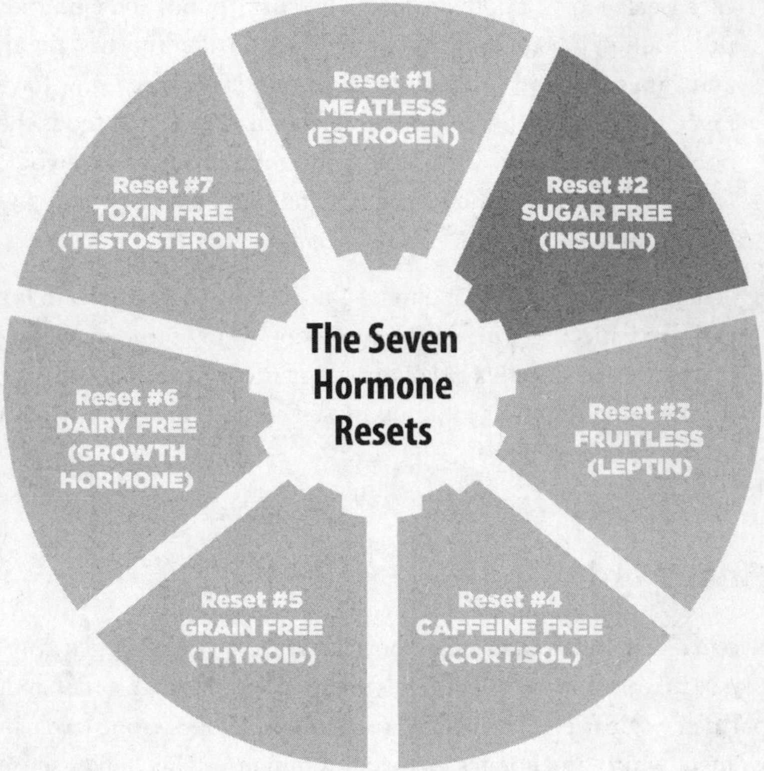

# The Seven Hormone Resets

Reset #1
MEATLESS
(ESTROGEN)

Reset #2
SUGAR FREE
(INSULIN)

Reset #3
FRUITLESS
(LEPTIN)

Reset #4
CAFFEINE FREE
(CORTISOL)

Reset #5
GRAIN FREE
(THYROID)

Reset #6
DAIRY FREE
(GROWTH
HORMONE)

Reset #7
TOXIN FREE
(TESTOSTERONE)

# CHAPTER 4

# Sugar Free

INSULIN RESET: *Days 4 to 6*

We all know the problem with sugar. It's addictive. It's bad for your teeth. It makes you lethargic, cranky, and enslaved. It feeds the bacteria in your gut that make you hang on to fat, which then makes you gain even more fat. But you might not understand that sugar is the main reason you can't fit into the form-fitting dress you wore a few years ago. It's not that you are eating too many calories and not exercising enough. It is far more likely that you can't zip the dress because you have insulin resistance, where your cells become numb to insulin. Why does this matter? Because insulin can control whether a calorie makes you fat. It's another important example of how hormones dictate what your body does with food. Current science suggests that a calorie of carbohydrate is more fattening than a calorie of protein or fat because of the effect on insulin. Too many of the wrong carbs cause insulin resistance. In fact, the solution to lasting weight loss is to maintain normal insulin levels.

Got your attention? Let me explain. Insulin is a hormone in charge of how you derive energy from the foods you eat. Your body runs on glucose, and insulin is one of the master switches. When serving you properly, insulin takes the glucose from the occasional cupcake you eat and stores it in the cells of the liver and muscles as glycogen—a storage form of glucose that can be broken down readily when you need fuel. You are filling up your tank with the gas it needs to run, and sometimes an aggregate of several thousand glucose molecules are kept in the glycogen storage space, like stacking Legos, depending on your fitness. But the catch is that you can only store a small amount of glycogen at any given time. When you eat a cupcake or two every day, there may not be room left in your tank to store the glucose as glycogen. Then insulin turns devious, transforming from a fat-*burning* hormone into a fat-*storage* hormone once the glycogen storage tank is full. Day in and day out, you are stuck converting carbohydrates into fat instead of using it for the fuel you desperately need, and storing the fat in your liver, waistline, and other organs. That's why so many women find themselves in a frustrating cycle of being 10 to 40 pounds (or more) overweight, lacking in energy, unable to zip the hot dress, and feeling hopeless.

Is insulin the reason you, like millions of other women, can't lose weight? Together we will figure it out. But I'm here to tell you that sometimes weight loss is a simple matter of resetting your insulin. I know many of you might say I'm asking the impossible. If you can't imagine life without your bars of chocolate stashed in your desk drawer, glove compartment, and purse, I understand. I've been there. But I implore you: you can do this for three days. And when you do, you'll find your sugar addiction broken and the pounds melting away.

## Self-Assessment

Insulin resistance is the most common hormonal reason I see in my medical practice for slow metabolism and weight gain in women. To see if you fit into this category, check off which symptoms apply to you or have occurred in the past six months.

☐ Do you crave sweet foods? Do sweet foods calm you down?

☐ Have you tried to stop eating sweets but found you couldn't? Is it difficult to stop eating carbohydrate-rich foods, such as chocolate, ice cream, or french fries?

☐ Have you been told your blood sugar is higher than normal, or do you know that it is greater than 85 mg/dL (milligrams per deciliter)?

☐ When you go without eating for more than three hours, do you feel shaky, anxious, or irritable?

☐ For women, is your waist measurement 35 inches or greater (at the belly button)? For men, greater than 40 inches?

☐ Do you have a body mass index greater than 25? (To calculate, see Measurement #2: Body Mass Index, Waist-to-Height Ratio, and Basal Metabolic Rate, page 27).

☐ Have you been told that you have polycystic ovary syndrome (PCOS), a condition that includes irregular periods, acne, increased hair growth, and sometimes infertility and cysts on the ovaries?

☐ Do you have difficulty losing weight? Do you gain weight easily, maybe even aggressively?

☐ When you skip a meal, do you feel fatigued and/or cranky?

☐ Do you exercise three times per week or less?

☐ Have you been told you have low HDL (good) cholesterol and/or triglycerides?

☐ Do you have high blood pressure (systolic greater than 140 or diastolic greater than 90)? Have you been told you have heart disease or atherosclerosis?

☐ Do you have a fasting insulin level that is greater than 5 µIU/mL (micro international units per milliliter)?

### Interpret Your Results

- **If you have five or more of these symptoms,** you are very likely insulin resistant, and I urge you to address this hormone imbalance quickly, since it puts you at significant risk for prediabetes and diabetes.

- **If you have four or fewer of these symptoms,** you might have insulin resistance, and I recommend asking your doctor for a blood (serum) test of your fasting glucose and insulin. Even better, request a two-hour glucose/insulin test.

You can reset your insulin pathway within seventy-two hours if you follow the rules. This is not just my opinion; it's based on rigorous science.[1] That's right, you can step into the grace of metabolic intelligence in a mere three days. You will train your body to be the fat-burning machine you've always wanted. Grace is your birthright, and what I've observed in twenty-plus years of medical practice is that it is given to humans who earn it. You can earn it too.

---

### From Dr. Sara's Case Files: Jeanette, Age Sixty

---

- *Started the Hormone Reset very depressed, barely sleeping, no energy, and anxious. "I felt like I was going to have a nervous breakdown."*
- *Lost 18 pounds in her first Hormone Reset*
- *Hardest reset was Sugar Free. "I used to be able to wipe out half a crumb cake. My sense of taste changed, and I now can barely eat a small piece."*
- *Lost another 18 pounds after she completed the program.*
- *Waist went from 36 to 31 inches; hips 38 to 36 inches.*
- *"I bought a glucometer and supplies expecting it to be a waste and was shocked that my fasting blood sugars were 100 to 114. Now I'm running around 85."*

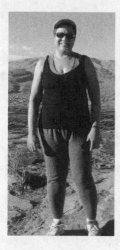 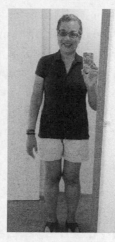

- Able to work with clinician to wean off her medications (amlodipine and chlorthalidone).
- Now: "I feel so much better. I can think clearly again. I feel energetic. I can't believe how different my life is. I'm just plain happy again."

## Meet Insulin

Hormones are a vital part of our body's cell-to-cell communication and response system. When that system breaks down, many problems occur. Eighty percent of the time that includes weight gain, according to a quantitative survey I've performed among my patients.

Insulin and its receptors fit together like a key fits into a lock. How do you know when your insulin hormones and receptors don't fit well? Here's an easy test: lift up your shirt and look at your belly. If yours could be mistaken for Jennifer Aniston's, your insulin is probably fine. If your stomach is spilling over your yoga pants (or you just prefer to wear yoga pants so that you don't have to squeeze into your jeans), it's time to reset your insulin so that it's in the target zone.

Insulin is the gatekeeper of many other hormones of metabolism, which is why I put the Sugar Free reset second, after the easy win of Meatless. High insulin leads to estrogen dominance, and it also raises testosterone too high, which may make weight-loss resistance worse. Additionally, insulin is a cousin to leptin, the hormone made in your fat cells that tells your body, "Darling, put down the fork." As I'll explain in chapter 5, leptin signals a sense of satisfaction while eating, and insulin resistance raises leptin levels, eventually leading to leptin resistance, which means you don't get the signal to stop eating. To correct the problem, you'll flip the switch on insulin, and you'll get additional benefits: you'll improve your estrogen even more than you achieved in our first reset (Meatless), plus you'll begin to reset your testosterone and leptin.

## Good Fats, Clean Proteins . . . Slow Carbs

In the Sugar Free reset, you will dramatically reduce sugar and eat a low-glycemic food plan. This has been shown to reset the lazy insulin receptor and to reset testosterone, which is a hormone that tends to rise with increased stress and insulin resistance.

I hate to tell you bread lovers, but carbohydrates are not essential to survival. The foods that are necessary are healthy fats (such as omega-3s) and clean proteins, which contain certain vital amino acids. But you would survive without carbohydrates.

That doesn't mean that you need to remove carbohydrates completely. Severe restriction can actually raise your reverse T3, a metabolic hormone that blocks your thyroid receptor (see chapter 7). Severe carb restriction may also raise stress hormones, such as cortisol (see chapter 6). Instead, you should be like Switzerland: in a neutral zone, where you eat enough carbs to prevent problems with your thyroid and cortisol, but not so many that you store more fat, which some call the "carb threshold."

When you start the Hormone Reset, I want to limit your selection to the slow-burning carbs that come from plants, included in your pound of vegetables per day, plus clean proteins, such as crustaceans, seafood, beans, small servings of nuts, and seeds. Become familiar with how many grams or ounces of carbs you're taking in. The neutral zone with carbohydrates varies from person to person, and it has a lot to do with your genetics and how insulin resistant you are, but the target is approximately 20 to 49 grams of slow-burning net carbs per day for weight loss.

Measuring your net carbs was discussed in chapter 2 (page 32): Take the total carbohydrate content of your food and subtract the fiber content. For instance, if you steam 6 ounces of asparagus and eat it, you're getting 6 grams of carbohydrates plus 6 grams of fiber. So, the net carbs are zero: 6–6 = 0.

See the following chart for more information.

## Net Carbohydrate Thresholds

| | |
|---|---|
| **<20g** | When you eat less than 20 grams of net carbs per day, you can enter ketosis, which can raise your cortisol and activate a thyroid blocker called reverse T3. |
| **20-49g** | Your goal is to eat 20 to 49 grams of net carbs per day, from plants. This will keep you out of ketosis but will reset your insulin. |
| **50-99g** | During Sustenance, you can experiment with eating more net carbs. Slowly increase to 50 to 99 grams. For me, 75 is my upper limit. |
| **>99g** | Eating more than 99 grams of net carbs per day tends to increase insulin resistance. |

When you're insulin resistant, you tend to have other hormonal problems, almost like the "buy one, get one free" deal at your local supermarket. High insulin levels make your ovaries secrete more testosterone. Your cells also produce more bad estrogens, and you become leptin resistant. Fortunately, when you start the three-day Sugar Free reset, the other fat-storage imbalances likewise improve.

In fact, a low-glycemic food plan also reduces testosterone and its related hormones by 20 percent, according to research from Australia.[2] In this study, a group of twelve men ate a low-glycemic-load food plan (25 percent energy from proteins and 45 percent from low-glycemic carbohydrates). Within seven days, their insulin improved and their testosterone dropped significantly, as measured by the free androgen index.[3]

Here's the best news: it's never too late, and I've never found a lost cause in my twenty-plus years of taking care of patients. It's my aim to meet you where you are and to move you forward slowly or quickly as you reset your hormone receptors.

## Sugar Addiction

Foods high in sugar trigger the reward centers of your brain. A perfect storm may occur in people who are vulnerable to food addiction: they eat sugar, resulting in high blood sugar and low dopamine in the brain. When they keep eating sugar, they develop problems with dopamine communication. They need more and more sugary foods to raise their dopamine and feel "normal," and they experience withdrawal symptoms when they remove sugar.

Women are twice as likely to be addicted to food as men.[4] Women tend to diet, restrict, and binge more than men, which seems to trigger the brain to overeat addictively. Interestingly, women with the greatest hormonal upheaval at perimenopause report the highest rates of food addiction.[5]

## Getting to Know Your Inner Saboteur

When I was a kid, I figured my discernment would improve as I got older. Then as I got older, I realized that my discernment isn't fancy:

I simply am able to distinguish my inner divine voice from my inner saboteur—the voice of my ego or of grasping.

For the next twenty-four hours, focus on your inner saboteur and its wily ways. Take some time to root out the mental and emotional obstacles, beliefs, and attitudes that may sabotage your success with the Hormone Reset. As you become more familiar with your inner saboteur, you learn there are many ways that voice shows up in your life. What does your inner saboteur say to you? When is the voice the loudest? Or is there some other way that you can become more intuitive about this aspect of yourself regarding food? To get you thinking, here is Doreen's example:

> "Mine has a theme song: 'You can start/restart tomorrow.' Now I know I needed a commitment to something bigger than myself. I don't let my inner saboteur set the schedule and play the tomorrow game." —*Doreen*

Noticing how your inner saboteur undermines you is the first step! Next, we will start the process of how to quiet the saboteur and then swap the harmful voice for faith, trust, ideologies, and convictions that are more aligned with your personal food code. What's fascinating is that most people don't even realize they have this inner voice until they slow down and listen. We are so sure these stories are true. I'm here to tell you that the saboteur is smart—but you are smarter! With a little introspection, you can start to tell your saboteur that you are sick of its stories and have chosen a truer path of intuitive health.

In *Emotional Freedom*, Judith Orloff, M.D., talks about that intuitive state between wakefulness and sleep when negative or spooky "waking dreams" can besiege you. She says you have the right to tell them to stop. "It's fine to ignore them or insist they desist, either inwardly or aloud," she writes.[6] Apply that same intelligence to your saboteur!

# The Problem of Insulin Resistance

Insulin is one of seven crucial hormones (estrogen, leptin, cortisol, thyroid, testosterone, and growth hormone are the others) that collectively determine your metabolism, or how fast or slow you burn calories. When your cells become resistant to insulin, your body is programmed to raise your insulin levels higher and higher. This is troubling because these hormones regulate your metabolism, and "higher and higher" hormones do not lead to a faster metabolism. In fact, chronically elevated hormone levels signal that your feedback loops have gone rogue.

When your hormones are elevated, your metabolism gets slower and slower, while you get fatter and fatter. This is why you may hear your girlfriends complaining that they've been restricting their food intake, exercising like crazy, and surviving on lettuce leaves without losing weight. The insidious hormone-resistance and biological-feedback loop is the root cause of most women's continued weight gain, belly fat, wrinkles, exhaustion, autoimmune disorders, inflammation, sugar cravings, and even chronic illness.

You may wonder why you're programmed to become insulin resistant when you overeat certain foods. Like many challenges, the tendency to raise insulin levels excessively and slow down metabolism comes from our ancestors' feast-or-famine livelihoods, when they had to be able to store excess energy at the time of feasting in order to survive a time of famine. Not only is the survival strategy of preparing for a famine no longer necessary, it backfires. As an achievement-oriented woman with significant drive, I can power my way through a situation and turn on a famine of my own creation. Put another way, I can produce insulin resistance in my own body simply by feeling overly stressed.

The only way to reverse this resistance and reprogram your hormonal levels is to repair and grow new hormone receptors.

This is an exciting idea that hasn't been fully explored in mainstream medicine for several reasons. Some of the data on hormone resistance are new. Some of the data on how food can reverse insulin resistance are ignored, in my opinion, because they rely on nutrition as the solution, and most medical schools teach very little nutrition. Personally, I had a total of about thirty minutes in my medical training. In other words, it's not intentionally omitted by your doctor; it's simply a lack of education and resulting prioritization. Finally, reversing insulin resistance with the way you eat, move, think, and supplement doesn't support the financial goals of Big Food and Big Pharma. Big Food wants you eating packaged foods, more carbohydrates than you need, and "hyperpalatable" foods (foods that have been engineered, with added fats, flavors, and additives, to become addictive). Big Pharma then wants your doctor to prescribe many fancy drugs for the problems that develop from eating a Big Food diet.

## WHEN INSULIN BECOMES THE OVERWHELMED BODYGUARD

*Food increases blood sugar. Insulin lowers it by escorting glucose, like a bodyguard, into three different places in your body. Insulin is a regulatory hormone, made in the pancreas, that causes cells to absorb glucose from the blood and take it to the liver, muscles, and fat tissue. When insulin is in good working form—not too high and not too low—it sends a small amount of glucose to your liver, a large amount to your muscles to use as fuel, and little to none to your fat storage. When you're a perfect hormonal specimen, your pancreas produces exactly the right amount of insulin to have your blood sugar softly rise and fall within a narrow range (fasting levels of 70 to 85 mg/dL).*

*But when you eat too much sugar, your pancreas slows down, and eventually, insulin becomes the overwhelmed bodyguard. Here's what wears out the bodyguard: eating too much sugar causes wild fluc-*

tuations, both too high and too low, in your blood sugar, and insulin can't keep up. As a result, your pancreas keeps making more and more insulin. Insulin levels rise chronically high, which is called insulin resistance. Blood sugar then stays high because very little glucose is escorted to the liver and muscles, and most is deposited as fat. In fact, your fat tissue can expand up to four times its size to accommodate the storage of glucose.

There are several ways you can reset insulin's bodyguard role without using drugs:

- **Eat foods that stabilize blood glucose,** i.e., clean proteins, slow-burning carbs, and healthy fats. This will lower your insulin levels into the target zone and is the most effective way to activate insulin (see the Sugar Free reset rules, page 88).
- **Exercise** so that your liver and skeletal muscles can store more glucose as glycogen and use it as fuel (see the Exercise section, page 94).
- **Take supplements** that help to sensitize your cells to insulin again, and rehab the bodyguard (see the Supplements section, page 92).

## The Science Behind Sugar Free

Let's follow the path of a bite of cupcake in order to understand the science of insulin and how it can get out of whack. Normally, you absorb the cupcake into your bloodstream as a sugar, such as glucose. An increase in your blood sugar level triggers your pancreas to make more insulin, which attaches to your cells and removes sugar from your blood so it can be used as energy. Initially, your insulin targets mainly muscle and liver cells.

When you have insulin resistance, your cells have a decreased capacity to respond to insulin. To compensate for the decreased sensitivity to insulin, your pancreas secretes more insulin to try to grab the attention of the worn-out cell receptors. Higher levels of insulin then create inflammation, make your blood sugar swing from high to low, and cause you to feel hungry soon after eating. When insulin remains high, you are no longer a lean, mean, fat-burning machine. Because your cells cannot absorb the glucose normally, your liver converts the glucose into fat.

Fortunately, insulin resistance is reversible. Even if you feel totally out of control with your sugar cravings, I can help you. That's because when you cut out sugar, your cravings will heal and your insulin will normalize. Make this important change for yourself.

Keep in mind that sugar is powerfully addictive.[7] I put sugar in the same category as addictive drugs like crack or heroin. Take Oreos, for example. One study from Connecticut showed that rats fed the iconic cookie liked it as much as cocaine and morphine.[8] When the rats ate Oreo cookies, the pleasure center of their brains, the nucleus accumbens, lit up like a Christmas tree—the same area in the brain that lights up with cocaine. Sugar and cocaine both stimulate the addictive part of the brain with a neurotransmitter called dopamine, known for its role in pleasure and satisfaction. Rats in the study even broke open the cookie to eat the sugary middle first. Still not sure if you're addicted to sugar? One study showed that 34 percent of people seeking weight loss are food addicts.[9]

Sugar substitutes fare no better. Indeed, one study suggests that saccharin is eight times more addictive than cocaine.[10]

## Sugar Free: The Three-Day Reset for Insulin

Let's start! Remember, the seventy-two-hour reset is a simple way to take care of the chronic symptoms that plague you, especially fat gain. Each cycle takes a mere three days to reverse and reset your body's hormone receptors. Of course, the Hormone Reset is a twenty-one-day program, so as you focus on each reset and tune into the changes that reset brings, you'll achieve the full benefits of the program by continuing each reset for the balance of the twenty-one days. The Sugar Free reset is one crucial piece of the puzzle.

My clinical experience has taught me that resetting your insulin is the single most important action you can take to lose excess fat. Perhaps you have been trying to lose weight for years, or even decades, leading you to feel hopeless, stuck, and desperate. You are not alone.

You need to cut the sugar. This includes all the usual suspects, such as cakes, cookies, muffins, and soda. If you think you can simply switch to another sweet, addictive substance, sorry again. "No sugar" includes sugar substitutes too, with the exception of stevia. Scrutinize labels because sugar lurks in the most unsuspected places and hides under various names. Look for grams of sugar. With this reset, you'll be aiming for no more than 15 grams per day, 10 less than the 25 grams per day currently recommended for women by the American Heart Association.

It's easier than it sounds. Research confirms that you can repair your insulin receptors in seventy-two hours. The seven resets of your Hormone Reset will resynchronize your entire system when performed sequentially and in aggregate.

## SUGAR FREE RULES: DO THESE EACH DAY

Follow these simple yet powerful rules to reset your insulin, and continue the rules you've already implemented from chapter 3 (Meatless):

1. **Eliminate sugar and sugar substitutes.** Avoid these because they raise your blood sugar: white table sugar, honey, agave, brown sugar, sucralose (Splenda), maple syrup, and molasses. The only sweetener that is permissible is stevia. Limit carbohydrates to only

the slow carbohydrates that don't spike your insulin, such as sweet potatoes, yams, pumpkin, and quinoa. Stay away from hidden sugars in ketchup, salad dressings, sauces, and packaged cereals. If sugar is one of the first six ingredients, avoid it. Stay off the liquid sugar, including soda, diet soda, juice, lemonade, and alcohol.

2. **Eat one pound of vegetables,** some cooked and some raw. For those of you who are losing steam around eating vegetables, I urge you to keep eating three to four cups (sixteen or more ounces) per day. For instance, eat a salad for breakfast (not as weird as you might think!) or make a frittata with eggs and spinach. Have a salad plus a serving or two of green vegetables at both lunch and dinner. That's seven servings! The easiest way to accomplish this task is to lightly steam a pot of vegetables, such as broccoli, mushrooms, asparagus, and red bell peppers, every few days and have them on hand to make a salad for lunch and dinner. Aim for low-glycemic vegetables with low starch, not corn (a fruit when fresh, and deemed a grain when dried) or other starchy vegetables. Choose vegetables that are dark, because dark vegetables are low in glycemic index and high in important nutrients. Often it's more affordable to have a box of organic vegetables delivered from your local farm, which is what I do. I take my greens (kale, collards, spinach) when they first arrive, chop them finely, and store them in a bag in the freezer. Then, as I steam my vegetables I add the greens near the end, or I add them to my salads or to my Hormone Reset shakes.

3. **Eat protein at each meal,** approximately 4 to 6 ounces of fish or chicken, beans, or quinoa. Fill up on legumes, especially the magical white kidney bean, which contains a carb blocker. Aim for a total of 75 to 125 milligrams of protein each day, which is approximately 25 to 45 grams at each of three meals.
   *Food List:* Lentils (fast cooking!), black beans, pinto beans, white kidney beans, fish (cod, salmon, mackerel, sardines), and free-range, pastured, or organic chicken.

4. **Eat at least every four to six hours.** If you feel like you always need a snack and frankly are willing to eat cardboard after three hours, that's a clear sign that you are insulin resistant, have blood sugar instability, and need the reset in this chapter! I do not recommend snacks unless absolutely necessary—the goal is to reset your insulin level. And if you feel like you need snacks, it might mean you're not getting enough protein at meals. If you feel hypoglycemic before four hours have elapsed between meals, drink 8 ounces of filtered water and set a timer for twenty minutes. Try one or more of the Cell to Soul Practice suggestions in any of the chapters 3 through 10. If twenty minutes elapse and you're still famished, eat ten almonds or walnuts.

5. **Eat one half-cup of low-glycemic fruit** (glycemic index 55 or less), such as berries, avocado, or olives. Banish all other fructose, including the high-glycemic fruits, such as bananas, mangos, and grapes—and wine!
   *Food List:* Avocado, berries, coconut, olives.

6. **Eat the highest quality, most nutrient-dense organic food** you can afford. Focus on low-glycemic index greens, such as kale, chard, dandelion greens, spinach, and collards.

7. **Eat probiotic foods.** Fermented foods contain natural probiotics, or healthy bacteria, that can take your health to the next level. Not only do they add good bacteria into your stomach and your gut, they're also powerhouses when it comes to detoxification, especially of heavy metals.[11] Nearly every culture has a version of a fermented food: yogurt, kefir, miso, and fermented vegetables, including sauerkraut, pickles, and kimchi.
   • *Kimchi.* In Korea, the average consumption of kimchi is 40 kilograms per year! The lactic acid that is produced during fermentation of kimchi stops the growth of bad bacteria and is useful in the prevention of conditions such as obesity, diabetes, yeast infections, urinary tract infections, and gastrointestinal cancers. One recent study showed that kimchi improved fasting

glucose and cholesterol levels.[12] Nutritionally, kimchi is low in calories and carbohydrates but contains high amounts of fiber, vitamins A and C, and minerals such as calcium and iron.

## SAMPLE MENU

Here is a suggested menu for resetting your insulin. For nutritional data, check out the Notes section.[13]

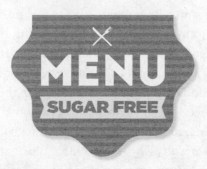

| BREAKFAST | 1 cup hot water (alkaline-forming) or herbal tea with lemon<br><br>2 egg whites plus 2 whole eggs cooked with 1 cup sliced green vegetables (asparagus, zucchini, kale, chard, arugula) |
| --- | --- |
| LUNCH | 1 cup sautéed greens (kale, chard, and spinach, or mustard, turnip, and beet greens) with 1 tablespoon organic, pastured ghee<br><br>6-ounce organic turkey burger, wrapped in romaine lettuce leaves or collard greens<br><br>Quick Green Tonic (see Recipes) with 1 tablespoon MCT oil |
| DINNER | 4 to 6 ounces cod, cut up and sautéed in 1 tablespoon red palm or coconut oil<br><br>6 ounces Brussels sprouts, sautéed in 1 tablespoon red palm or coconut oil<br><br>1 to 2 cups salad with 1 tablespoon avocado or olive oil and 1 tablespoon red wine vinegar to taste |

## Supplements

When it comes to your insulin reset, I agree with Hippocrates: food is your best medicine. However, exercise and supplements can help you get to the next level in resetting this important hormone by going sugar free. As a board-certified physician, I don't rely on anecdotes when it comes to supplements. The supplements I recommend have data to back up taking them. A list of insulin-resetting supplements, including alpha lipoic acid, berberine, chromium, fenugreek, cinnamon, bitter melon, probiotics, vanadium, and others, and a summary of the science can be found at www.HormoneReset.com/bonus. Yet the supplement I find most helpful in the Sugar Free reset is one that addresses sugar cravings with a combination of L-tyrosine and 5-HTP. I love tyrosine because it helps women focus and reduces cravings. It's an amino acid—the building block of protein—and it gives you the clarity and energy that people seek from sugar, but without the side effects. It has a precursor to dopamine, the brain chemical of focus and pleasure. It has been shown to help in reducing stress hormones. 5-HTP is also an amino acid, and a precursor to serotonin and melatonin, which are happy brain chemicals. I recommend a dose of tyrosine 500 to 1,000 milligrams, and 5-HTP 50 to 100 milligrams, and both should be taken one hour before breakfast and lunch.

## Cell to Soul Practice

My patients know to expect more than a signed prescription when they come to me. I've listened to thousands of women tell me that they feel overwhelmed, overworked, and totally stressed out. The connection is undeniably clear in my practice, and science backs me up: the vicious cycle of chronic unmanaged stress feeds insulin resistance. That means we need to replace your vicious cycle of stress with a virtuous cycle of self-care. This involves not only the food you eat but also the thoughts you think.

As a yoga teacher, I'm all for cultivating positive emotions and deep relaxation. I think it's a crucial part of maintaining a healthy body and mind. But my vision for you goes beyond relaxation to a state known as "coherence," a term essential to the philosophy of HeartMath, a nonprofit research and educational institute in Santa Cruz, California.

Coherence is a powerful physiological state that moves beyond relaxation and promotes optimal healing. When you reach this state, you have the ability to transform negative states like anger, stress, depression, and anxiety. When you attain coherence, you'll be relaxed but energized and aware, highly responsive, flexible, in the flow, and in the zone—that is, the normal zone of optimal cortisol, glucose, and insulin.

Science shows that the best way to reset stress is by synchronizing the two halves of the nervous system: the sympathetic (fight or flight) and the parasympathetic (rest and digest) to reach coherence. HeartMath has shown that coherence can significantly lower cortisol and reduce blood sugar.

Here is a practice to create quick coherence by applying a version of the Institute of HeartMath's methods.

## Quick Coherence

### Step One: Heart Focus

Bring your focus to your heart in the center of your chest.

### Step Two: Heart-Focused Breathing

Imagine your breath is flowing in and out of your heart. Take slow, steady deep breaths: inhale for five seconds and let your belly gently expand, and then exhale for five seconds. Allow your belly to softly contract toward your spine. Continue with this pattern for several minutes. You will feel much calmer and grounded.

### Step Three: Heart Feeling

Activate a positive feeling by remembering a time when you felt peaceful and centered inside (with a loved one, a pet, a time in nature, listening to your favorite music, etc.). Once you activate this feeling, stay for ten breaths. Continue to activate the positive feeling, and slowly begin to feel how your body and heart soak up the feeling.

## Exercise

When you are resetting your insulin pathway, you need to burn some calories with exercise daily to improve the benefits. I recommend the Hormone Reset Burst 7, during which you exercise at your usual pace (walk, jog, or ride a bike) for five minutes to warm up, then sprint at your highest effort for thirty seconds, then recover at your usual pace for two minutes. Repeat this for a total of seven cycles of thirty-second bursts. This form of exercise has been shown to lower insulin and raise growth hormone, an important "fountain of youth" hormone of metabolism described in chapter 8.

## Test Yourself

I recommend that you perform a fasting blood sugar test each morning to track your progress. While it takes a bit of practice, I strongly encourage you to learn how to test your blood sugar and use it as important feedback (see Measurement #6: Blood Sugar, page 30).

If you find that your blood sugar is normal (i.e., between 70 and 85 mg/dL), test yourself once per week and measure several post-prandial blood sugars. (Use the same technique to check your blood glucose two hours after a meal.)

If the idea of pricking your finger raises your stress hormones, ask your health-care professional to measure your fasting glucose and insulin at your local laboratory. Once again, you're looking for the optimal range for fasting glucose between 70 and 85 mg/dL, and fasting insulin of 5 µIU-mL. Your clinician may prefer to order a more thorough test called the oral glucose tolerance test (OGTT), which is tedious but more accurate for diagnosing patients with prediabetes or diabetes.

I've listed the normal and optimal ranges for tests related to insulin resistance (see Resources, page 291). Your doctor was probably taught to obey the mainstream "normal" ranges, which are derived by your laboratory and include the values for 95 percent of the population (the highest 2.5 percent and lowest 2.5 percent are excluded). In other words, to paraphrase acupuncturist and author Chris Kresser, these "normal" values are just common, not optimal. Since at least one in three Americans have insulin resistance, I want you to set a new goal of being in the "optimal" range, indicated in the third column of the table.

Record all blood sugars in your journal. Remember, even normal-weight individuals have problems with unstable blood sugar. I have found that women reverse prediabetes rapidly by following my Sugar Free rules, and the numbers prove it: the average fasting blood sugar dropped from 104 to 83 mg/dL, which is normal!

## Notes from Hormone Resetters

"I eliminated my sugar cravings! Additionally I have found that I respond to stress much differently. I feel it, notice it, and move on from it. Stress no longer has a grip on me. Freedom from both sugar and my stress response was a change I was hoping for, and it happened so seamlessly." —*Sophia*

"Exactly what I needed to break my cycle of food cravings. I suspected that caffeine and sugar were triggering an unhappy and unhealthy cycle for me, but now I know without a doubt. It is a wonderful feeling to let go of some emotional attachments to food, stop the craving cycle, shed some toxic fat, and feel anxiety get replaced by calm." —*Kasie*

"Scale says I'm down nearly 10 pounds. Sugar-withdrawal headaches seem to be gone, and most important, I feel . . . happier! Now I need to work on sleep!" —*Jennifer*

"Sugar is my nemesis, so I was shocked when I woke up feeling better than I have in the last two years! So much energy and very clear thinking, even felt like running again. Happy day!" —*Amy*

## Final Word

I'm excited for you to go sugar free and start resetting your insulin pathway. With this evidence-based way to lose weight for good, you'll stop suffering from the vicious cycles of wild blood sugar swings, sugar cravings, and increased belly fat. I believe you'll discover this is one of your most important steps toward your Hormone Reset.

When you're insulin resistant, you tend to have other hormonal problems. Your cells also produce more bad estrogens, and you become leptin resistant. High insulin levels make your ovaries secrete more testosterone than is healthy. (Remember, imbalanced testosterone keeps you from shedding the pounds. You want your testosterone to be just right: not too high and not too low.) Fortunately, when you start the three-day Sugar Free reset, the other fat-storage imbalances likewise improve.

I've learned over the years that you need to *want* the things that are good for you, even if they're hard. You may find it difficult to live without your nightly glass of white wine or after-dinner ice cream. But when you realize that you feel more energized and lose weight faster, I think you'll be motivated. Your body is the vessel of your soul, and some folks—like myself—consider it your sacred duty to feed your body and soul the best nutrients. If food is information for your DNA, sugar feeds your body the wrong information. I'm not saying you should deprive yourself of a small piece of your child's birthday cake or a piece of dark chocolate after a nice dinner. But daily consumption of refined sugar is equivalent to smoking two packs of cigarettes per day. It causes diabetes and prediabetes, which results in a fate that may include heart disease, high blood pressure, and cancer.

Even with all of my urging to banish sugar and refined carbohydrates, I want you to go easy on yourself if you slip. Ambitious women tend to hold themselves to an impossible standard of perfection. To paraphrase a favorite meme from Harry Truman: imperfect action trumps perfect inaction. If you backslide, take notice, but get right back on the path.

When you look at the long-term picture instead of settling for instant gratification, you create integrity. You may or may not believe in God or prefer to consider this concept more generally as "Source" or "Highest Self," but my point is the same: food is your portal to integrity in many other areas in your life, including your mind, body, spirit, finances, and relationships. When you make the choice to do what it takes to stay healthy, you are sending your body a powerful message that it deserves the best.

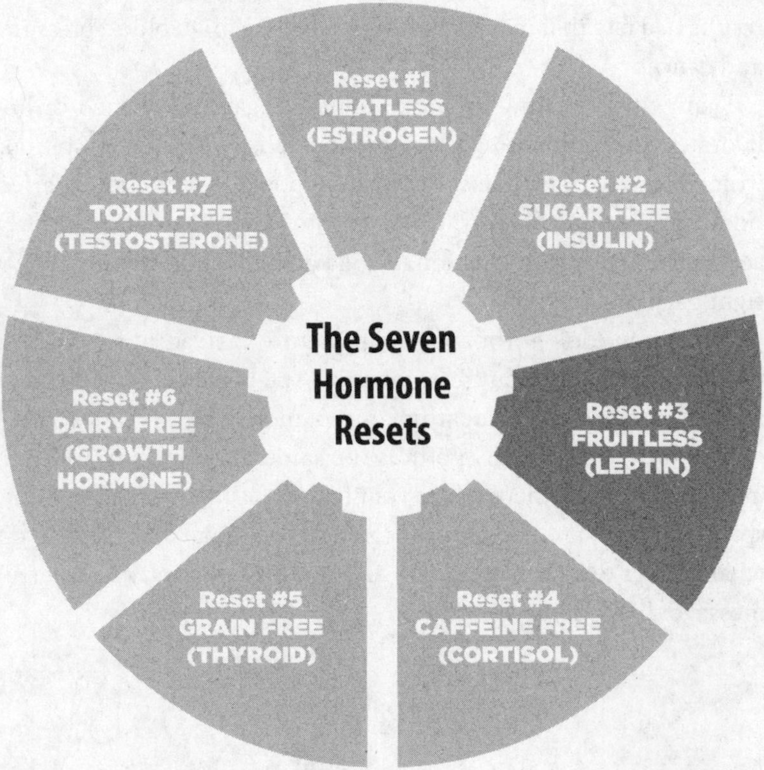

The Seven Hormone Resets

Reset #1
MEATLESS
(ESTROGEN)

Reset #2
SUGAR FREE
(INSULIN)

Reset #3
FRUITLESS
(LEPTIN)

Reset #4
CAFFEINE FREE
(CORTISOL)

Reset #5
GRAIN FREE
(THYROID)

Reset #6
DAIRY FREE
(GROWTH
HORMONE)

Reset #7
TOXIN FREE
(TESTOSTERONE)

# CHAPTER 5

# Fruitless

Now that you've done the hardest work of going meatless and sugar free in the last two resets, you're ready to restrict your use of fructose—the form of sugar that gives fruits, honey, sports drinks, and most sodas their sweet taste. I promise, this reset is easier! The good news is that when you put these three resets together, you've got the winning combination to get the three most important metabolic hormones activated to support you: estrogen, insulin, and leptin.

Maybe you're in love with your stash of dried apricots, which contain seventeen times the amount of fructose as fresh apricots. Fructose is the sugar that's naturally found in fruit, but it is also added to processed foods for taste and preservation—you may know one form as high-fructose corn syrup.

Fructose consumption is at an all-time high in the American diet, and it is linked to problems with insulin and another hormone called leptin, which is in charge of hunger. When you're overweight and/ or experience blood sugar issues, fructose may become a problem when calorie intake is too high. In fact, fructose is 73 percent sweeter than table sugar,[1] which makes it highly palatable and encourages overeating. Plus it's processed differently in the body. How much fructose is too much is subject to debate and probably depends on your current metabolism, what you eat (and overeat), genetics, how much you exercise, and your fitness level.

In my experience with patients, I have found 20 grams or less per day is ideal for a reset. I'll show you how to accomplish that in this chapter.

Why limit fructose? You're probably consuming too much because 75 percent of foods have sugar added in various forms, and some experts argue that it's the primary reason you're fat.[2] When you eat small amounts of fructose and your blood sugar is normal, you're okay. But if you eat too much, your liver can't process the fructose fast enough for the body to use it as fuel. Instead, your body starts converting the fructose into fats, sending them off into the bloodstream as triglycerides, and depositing them as fat in the liver and elsewhere in your belly.[3] Other issues with fructose overload include insulin resistance,[4] leptin resistance,[5] and cognitive decline.[6]

Fructose excess is like the biggest slide at the water park on a hot summer day. When there are too many kids on line, it gets backed up. Then kids get impatient and start cutting the line, wandering away, and jumping in the pool anyway.

The result? *Total chaos*, and in the body, it means *you get fat.*

Are you having problems with the water park in your body; that is, fructose excess and, by extension, leptin resistance? Let's find out by continuing our detective work to see if leptin is your dominant hormone imbalance.

## Self-Assessment

Take this self-assessment to see if you might be eating too much fructose and having a problem with leptin, an important hormone that regulates your body fat. Do you have or have you experienced in the past six months . . .

☐ A strong, sometimes insatiable appetite?

☐ Binge eating, especially after five P.M.? Eating after seven P.M. or within three hours of going to bed?

☐ A tendency to skip breakfast or wait an hour or longer after rising in the morning to eat?

☐ A love of drinking fruit juices or sodas, more than one serving per day?

☐ Excess weight or obesity (a body mass index over 25)? Count this item twice if you're 30 or more pounds overweight.

☐ Menopausal weight gain, especially at your waist?

☐ Increased fat in the skin covering your triceps muscles, sometimes affectionately known as "kimono arms"?

☐ A diagnosis of metabolic syndrome or insulin resistance (more than five symptoms listed at the beginning of chapter 4, page 77)?

☐ Weird or profuse sweating patterns compared with ten or twenty years ago?

☐ Fatigue after exercise and difficulty recovering completely?

☐ Joint problems—painful joints, joint destruction, bursitis, arthritis—or your doctor has suggested knee, hip, or shoulder surgery?

☐ High reverse T3 (RT3)? (This is a thyroid hormone, increased in leptin resistance, which blocks thyroid function.)

☐ High triglycerides, or you know them to be greater than 100 mg/dL?

### Interpret Your Results

- **If you have five or more of these symptoms,** you are *very likely* leptin resistant, and I urge you to address this hormone imbalance in this reset, since it puts you at significant risk for overeating, obesity, prediabetes, and diabetes. If leptin is the culprit, we'll lower it by cutting back on fructose in this chapter, and you'll lose weight.

- *If you have four or fewer of these symptoms or are unsure,* I recommend restricting fructose as described in this chapter and noticing the effect on your mood and weight.

According to the U.S. Department of Agriculture, compared with the 1950s, we eat 30 pounds more fruit annually.[7] Furthermore, the fruit has been bred by corporate farming to contain increasing amounts of fructose. Today, 200 calories of raw apple contain 25 grams of fructose—far more than the trace amount my great-grandmother consumed in an apple a hundred years ago.[8] Are we simply eating too much freaky fruit?

Ultimately, when you overconsume the wrong carbs, fructose can further impair your biochemistry. In fact, it's worse for your health than other sugars. In this chapter, you'll discover the powerful connection between fructose and leptin resistance, which dulls your appetite, regulates your hunger, and determines (together with insulin) how fast you burn fat.

When you overeat fructose, your leptin levels rise excessively—not only do you get fat but you feel ravenous too. My great-grandmother and her peers consumed about 15 grams of fructose per day in wild fruit, packaged in sufficient fiber, which created a serene, well-organized water park. Now the national average intake of fructose is more than triple that amount, and it's higher in adolescents.[9] Our DNA is not designed to handle these excessive amounts, so the extra fructose makes the kids go bonkers and misbehave, leptin levels rise, and mayhem erupts in the water park and on your bathroom scale. The truth is that fructose is not just a guilty pleasure; it's a public health menace that's making and keeping you fat. That's why eliminating fructose can lead to transformative changes in a very short time.

## A Sweet Cheat Sheet

Getting confused about the kinds of sugars? The following figure is a quick sugar guide, which is also summarized here. Note that the shared suffix of "-ose" means "sugar" or "carbohydrate."

- *Glucose* is found in sap and fruit, and it doesn't taste that sweet, so it's attached to fructose before being added to food as a sweetener.

- *Fructose*, or fruit sugar, is about twice as sweet as glucose. On its own, it causes malabsorption in many people, so it's attached to glucose when used as a sweetener for food and drinks.

- *Sucrose* is white table sugar. It contains one molecule of fructose connected to one molecule of glucose.

## Types of Sugar

| Monosaccharide (simple sugar) | |
|---|---|
| Glucose | • Found in sap and fruits<br>• Absorbed in small intestine, and 85 percent released into blood (remaining 15 percent leaks back into gut) |
| Fructose | • Found in fruits, honey, and green plants<br>• Sweeter than glucose<br>• Approximately 60 percent of the adult population has a limited ability to absorb fructose, and it gets stored as fat<br>• Commonly consumed as high-fructose corn syrup in breads, candy, cakes, cookies, ice creams, beverages, and processed foods<br>• Carbonated cola contains about 30 grams of fructose |
| Disaccharide (double sugar) | |
| Sucrose | • Ordinary table sugars found in juices, fruits, and roots<br>• Derived from one glucose molecule and one fructose molecule |

# Leptin 101

When you're healthy, with an ideal body mass index and normal fat composition, leptin is nature's appetite suppressant. When you've had enough to eat, leptin signals your brain to stop eating. I think of leptin as the hormone that says, "Enough. You're satisfied."

Unfortunately, when you are overweight (that is, your body mass index is greater than 25, which is the ratio of your weight to your height), your fat cells produce excess leptin. Your receptors for leptin can't keep up with the feedback loop or restore stability (known as homeostasis). You'd think more leptin would quell your appetite; in fact, the opposite happens. In the life-is-not-fair department, when your brain gets bombarded with leptin signals from too many fat cells, it shuts down from being overwhelmed. The result: leptin levels keep rising, receptors stop functioning—so your body doesn't get the leptin signal, and you don't feel full; you keep eating the wrong foods in an addictive pattern, and you keep gaining weight. Your body becomes leptin resistant—just as you can become insulin resistant. Cells in your liver, pancreas, fat, and brain are numb to the normal signals from the hormone. While your body is trying valiantly to make the necessary physiological corrections, you keep stuffing the wrong food into your mouth, hoping that it all will work itself out.

It's true: nearly all women who are overweight are stuck in a false state of perceived starvation, driven by leptin resistance. Even normal-weight women can have a problem with leptin, a problem known as being "skinny fat."

In my practice, I found that many of my patients were leptin resistant. They had a "hunger hormone" problem, not a problem of willpower. Leptin resistance is at the heart of carbohydrate cravings, increased hunger, and overeating—and paradoxically it results in your brain thinking that you're starving. It's like a broken thermostat. Your system keeps sensing the room is cold, even when it's hot. When it's functioning optimally, leptin can be a dieter's best friend because it normalizes appetite and reverses fat storage. But when it's not, it can become your worst enemy.

## The Science of Leptin

Leptin is the gatekeeper of your fat. Made in your fat cells, leptin regulates your feeling of satiety and your lean body mass. When you eat, leptin is produced in and released from your fat cells and then travels in the blood to your brain, where under normal circumstances it tells your hypothalamus (the part of your brain in charge of appetite) that you're full and can stop eating. But when your metabolism is broken and leptin isn't working properly, the wires between the gut and the brain are crossed. If you are overweight, rather than responding to higher levels of leptin by having your brain say "Enough," you find that the feeling of satiety doesn't happen. The best way to bring your leptin under control, so that it regulates appetite and fat storage the way nature intended, is to cut back on fructose and eat more clean proteins—and the benefit is that you burn more fat and feel full when consuming appropriate food quantities.

"Leptin" comes from the Greek word *leptos*, which means "thin," but when you're leptin resistant, the opposite happens: you become fatter. Leptin is insulin's sibling, and the two hormones work in tandem. You healed your insulin in the Sugar Free reset and now we'll heal your leptin in this reset.

## The Science Behind Fruitless

When I was a little girl and sick with a cold, I'd go to my grandmother's home while my mom worked. She let me watch her soap operas with her while she made orange juice from a can and poured me glass after glass, telling me it would give me vitamin C and help me feel better. As an adult, I learned that vegetables are a far better source of vitamin C and that two glasses of orange juice deliver about 20 grams of fructose. Perhaps it's the synthetic version of fructose that has ruined the ability of your body to process fructose. Until we fix your broken metabolism, we need to limit how much fructose you are consuming, because the dose makes the poison.

## How Leptin Resistance Ravages Your Body

In order to make your leptin work properly, your body needs to move it around freely. However, when your triglycerides are high, they block the leptin message in the brain. It's like loud music. Triglycerides keep your brain from being wise about food; the music is blaring. The only way to let the leptin move freely around your body is to lower your triglycerides, ideally to less than 50 mg/dL. However, a good start is first lowering them to less than 100 mg/dL.

Additionally, leptin resistance affects your immune and reproductive systems. When your immunity suffers, chronic inflammation develops. Leptin is a major player in the low-grade inflammation that won't turn off in people who are overweight or obese. Leptin resistance also impairs fertility and weakens your bones.

A leptin imbalance can cause joint pain and damage because too much leptin accelerates the breakdown of cartilage in your joints. The level of leptin in your blood corresponds to the level in your joints: the more leptin, the more potential joint damage.

The link between fructose, insulin resistance, leptin resistance, and liver problems is strong, but we are early in our understanding of why. While we still need randomized trials to show that fructose is the cause, evidence is mounting that you should stay away from liquid sugar, including juice, as well as any source of fructose that is not high in fiber. That means avoiding soda (even diet soda), sports drinks, bread, cereal, energy bars, flavored yogurt, and condiments.

Here are other factors that cause and/or worsen leptin resistance:

- *Too much fructose.* Eating excess fructose (over 20 grams per day) puts you at greater risk of leptin resistance because fructose is metabolized by the liver, an important regulator of your appetite and weight.[10] I'll teach you which foods contain fructose, and during this reset, you will stop eating them.

- *Bad circadian rhythm.* Leptin may get out of balance when you disrupt your delicate but incredibly important circadian rhythm by becoming addicted to caffeine, alcohol, or sugar. Eliminating these substances allows your body to get back to its natural rhythm.

- *Sleep debt.* Your leptin is also affected when you build up a sleep debt, the cumulative effect of not getting enough sleep.[11] Studies show a link between weight gain, lack of sleep, and insulin resistance.[12] Furthermore, sleep debt leads to dietary indiscretion and weight gain in women because you're too tired to make wise food choices.[13] In other words, get that solid seven to nine hours that your body really needs. Regardless of your ability to seemingly function on less sleep, odds are that you need it: only 3 percent of the population has a gene allowing them to function well on less sleep. Get over being a type A woman, says Arianna Huffington, cofounder of *The Huffington Post,* in a 2011 TED talk. After fainting from exhaustion and breaking her cheekbone, she has become an evangelist for getting a good night's sleep. Turn off the television, take a warm bath, read a relaxing book, and make a commitment to going to bed earlier.

When you lose weight, insulin resistance and leptin resistance can resolve. But you may continue to stay sensitive to these important metabolic hormones even if you regain weight.[14] That's why resetting your hormones using the seventy-two-hour method is such a critical piece of your weight-loss strategy.

# FRUCTOSE: The Scorecard

## PRO

- Fruit is probably fine if your metabolism is healthy, but choose wild fruit that's low in fructose, such as blueberries picked in the summer in Alaska.
- Amount of fructose you can tolerate depends on genetic variants as well as fitness training.
- Diabetes? Eating fruits and vegetables may be associated with a lower risk of diabetes, but the data is stronger with vegetables.
- Overeating fruit is unlikely to break your metabolism, but once broken (you're overweight or fat), too much fruit may become a problem.

## CON

- Excess fructose linked to greater risk of blood sugar problems, as indicated by weight gain, diabetes, and metabolic syndrome.
- Fruit changed in the past century. In 1900, we ate 15 grams per day of fructose; now we average 55 grams per day for adults and 73 grams for adolescents.
- Not all carb-based foods are the same; perhaps high-fructose corn syrup and fruit juices, which lack fiber, are the true villains.
- Fruit juice consumption is linked to a greater risk of diabetes in women.
- Dried fruit has more in common with candy: two hundred calories of dried apricots contain 10 grams of fructose. Raisins? 20 grams.
- Excess fructose consumption leads to "de novo lipogenesis," roughly translated as fat deposition.
- Our Paleo ancestors didn't eat fruit daily; they ate fruit in season, unlike what's recommended by mainstream nutritionists.
- Rats overfed fructose took one week to develop metabolic syndrome; evidence in humans is less conclusive, but there's a link between high fructose intake and increased belly fat and insulin.

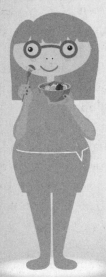

Fructose is potentially risky if you have blood sugar problems. It's the number one source of sugar in our diet, and it's a molecule responsible for our addiction to sweet foods. The rise in fructose consumption is highly correlated with obesity, diabetes, and a liver problem called nonalcoholic fatty liver disease, which now affects one in three Americans. Yet I want to be careful not to demonize fruit across the board for all people. The issue is more nuanced.

Here's the problem as I see it: vegetables are the best medicine when it comes to healing hormone imbalances that cause broken metabolism. When experts tell women to eat seven to nine servings of fresh fruits and vegetables each day, many women who are overweight simply eat more fruit—and don't lose weight. That's because existing blood sugar problems, found in half of U.S. women, make fructose a problem. If you're a normal eater and lean, with no blood sugar problems, fruit is fine. For the rest of us, there are shades of gray when it comes to eating whole fruit, avoiding juice, and limiting total fructose. When you heal your metabolism, you can eat more fructose without causing weight gain, but let's review cases for and against fructose. (For citations, go to www.HormoneReset .com/bonus.)

### ARE YOU "SKINNY FAT" AND UNHEALTHY?

*If you're normal in weight, you may not be as healthy as you think. You might be a "skinny fat" person, a term used to describe the one in four normal-weight individuals with increased fat mass. Skinny fat is a problem of body composition: you have too much fat mass relative to muscle mass, and the fat could be making you sick.*

*Let me give you a visual. Skinny fat women look thin but have very little muscle definition. They may look good in a T-shirt, but when naked, the belly appears doughy. When you touch their skin, you sink into fat rather than feel the firmness of muscles in the space between their skin and bones. They are thin people who are actually high in fat*

mass, especially around the belly, and low in muscle mass. They are
at risk of the same kinds of diseases as obese people: prediabetes,
diabetes, heart disease, and metabolic syndrome.

The clunky official medical term for this is "normal weight obesity,"
which means "Honey, you may look normal from the outside, but
inside you have too many fat cells (especially at your waist) and not
enough muscle mass." Shockingly, skinny fat people may have double
the mortality rates of overweight or obese people.[15]

How do you know if this is you? An optimal body fat range is 20 to
28 percent (14 to 20 percent for athletes). Fit and lean women have
a body fat of 21 to 24 percent; 32 percent and higher is considered
obese, according to the American Council on Exercise.[16]

Just as both fat and thin people can have insulin resistance, both fat
and thin people can have leptin resistance, although rates are higher
when you're obese.

Inflammation is at the root of why skinny fat, overweight, and
obese people have altered chemistry. It's like a bad neighborhood for
the cells of your body—and excess fructose adds more violence and
despair. People with minimal inflammation tend to be lean, happy,
and in hormonal balance.

Women are more likely to be skinny fat than men, because we have
fat cells that are more relentless; we're wired to stay chubby so we
can be fertile. We all know that we are targeted by the cultural ideals
of thinness, and that makes some women restrict food excessively
and become skinny fat. As we've learned, this is also damaging to
your metabolic fire.

In summary, wellness is more than just about ideal body weight;
it's about achieving your best lean body mass and health.

When insulin and leptin and their receptors are optimal, you have
normal lean body mass and are fit. The muscle and fat are evenly
distributed. You are fine with showing off your upper arms and belly.
You don't cower at the thought of going to the beach or wearing a
sleeveless dress. But when your receptors are having trouble mating,

*you could experience health problems, poor metabolism, and "sick fat"—even if you are technically skinny. What's a girl to do? Follow my twenty-one-day Hormone Reset so that you can lose fat mass and, over time, aim for an optimal body fat range.*

———————

**THE HUNGER GAMES: HOW LEPTIN MAKES YOU HUNGRY**

*Leptin resistance causes hunger in two extremes of the range: high and low. Your hypothalamus in your brain interprets both low leptin (less than 4 ng/mL) and high leptin (greater than 10 ng/mL) as an indication of starvation and revs up your appetite. Levels of leptin in your blood rise with your body fat.*[17] *When leptin is high, your brain is convinced you're starving, even though your body may have more than enough food. You feel hungry but never satisfied when you eat. So, you keep eating and keep gaining weight. Sound familiar? While leptin is playing a cruel joke on your body, insulin works against you too. Because insulin blocks effective action of leptin in the hypothalamus of your brain, high insulin begets high leptin. So, your brain believes you are starving and encourages you to overeat. This is another example of how normal physiology can turn against you. But it doesn't have to be a repeat performance playing out on an endless loop. Carefully following the Hormone Reset can help bring you back into a state of balance.*

———————

## Your Belly Fat and You

Obesity is a fat accumulation problem, and the locus is your belly. When you experience a roller coaster of blood sugar extremes, and you make too much insulin and estrogen, you deposit extra fat in your belly, mostly deep visceral fat. (You also deposit subcutaneous fat, which is just beneath the skin—the main point is that belly fat is worse for you.) Not only do you increase your waist size but you also deposit more fat inside your organs, such as in the liver, pancreas, kidneys, and intestines. Remember, fat cells manufacture excessive leptin, which floods the brain until it short-circuits and refuses to receive the satiety signal when you're full. It's like the assembly line gone awry: your brain can't keep up with the supply.

Fat deposits elsewhere—at your hips, buttocks, and arms—are not as dangerous as visceral or belly fat. They don't make high levels of leptin and other potentially harmful chemicals.

Your visceral fat, however, is a 24/7 factory that produces toxic chemicals called adipokines (inflammatory mediators made in your fat cells), which cause harm to your metabolism, hormone receptors, immune system, and joints. A protective hormone, adiponectin, which manages fat, may be abnormally low in obese people with certain genetic tendencies and further contributes to the dysfunctional pattern and increased inflammation.

---

### From Dr. Sara's Case Files: Cathy, Age Fifty-Three

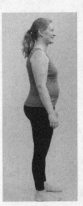
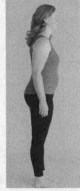

- *Lost 17 pounds, beginning in the prep phase!*
- *Normalized leptin to 4.5 ng/mL.*
- *Raised cortisol from low (6.7) to normal (12.0).*
- *Reduced inflammation (high sensitivity c-reactive protein reduced from 2.2 to 1.5, and homocysteine dropped from 9.7 to 8.7)*

- *"I would tell my friend this is a doctor-led [program] with a lot of science behind it. It increased my energy levels to better than I've had in more than three years, and I lost very stubborn pounds along the way."*

---

## FODMAPS

Up to 60 percent of adults cannot digest fructose properly and get gassy from certain rapidly fermentable (gas-producing) carbohydrates, such as the fructose in apples, apricots, cherries, mangos, nectarines, peaches, pears, and watermelon. The problem with absorption occurs in the small intestine, and researchers have found it extends beyond fructose to other related carbohydrates. Collectively, these problem foods are known as FODMAPS, which stands for "fermentable oligosaccharides (fructans and galactans), disaccharides (lactose), monosaccharides (fructose), and polyols (such as sorbitol, mannitol, and xylitol)." When these foods adversely affect you, it's called "FODMAPS malabsorption."

When this happens, these carbs travel to the large intestine, where they ferment, create gas, distend the bowel, cause bloating and pain, and may affect movement of food through the gut (i.e., diarrhea or constipation).[18] One of the reasons that many people don't digest fructose well is that the transport mechanism across the bowel wall is slow and low in capacity.

Healthy individuals can absorb about 25 to 50 grams of fructose, and most people with FODMAPs malabsorption difficulty can digest less than 25 grams during a meal. You can assess your ability to absorb FODMAPs with a hydrogen breath test. Limiting FODMAPs has been shown to help prevent gas, irritable bowel syndrome, and other functional gut disorders. People with fructose malabsorption have altered gastrointestinal motility, a mucosal biofilm, and altered microbiome.

---

# Fruitless: The Three-Day Reset
# for Leptin

Restricting fructose improves both insulin resistance and leptin levels.[19] While I don't believe in a single magic bullet, I have seen amazing results when my patients get their leptin levels in check by eliminating fructose and increasing their protein intake, especially within thirty minutes of getting out of bed in the morning. Not only do they lose fat, normalize their appetite, and feel relieved, they stop blaming themselves for their weight gain.

Our goal together in this reset is to normalize leptin. When leptin is signaling normally in your body, you stop getting a feel-good dopamine hit from the brain after you've taken in the right amount of food. (Dopamine is the brain chemical of pleasure and satisfaction.) You put down your fork when you're full. But when you are resistant to leptin, food doesn't stop tasting scrumptious, regardless of quantity—and that's why many overweight people find it nearly impossible to stop eating. When you reset leptin, you suppress dopamine and food stops tasting addictively good. When you do Fruitless, you reset your relationship to food, and that cupcake stops calling your name.

For long-term fat loss, you must flip the hunger switch—starting now. Just as you need to take a break from work to take a vacation, your receptors need a vacation from the wrong foods you've been throwing at them. In the following Fruitless reset guide, your first task is to upgrade your food choices so that you clear fructose from your system. I'm excited to show you how!

## FRUITLESS RULES: DO THESE EACH DAY

To get leptin back on your team, follow these rules:

1. **Start your day with protein.** Eat protein within thirty minutes of awakening, which reduces cravings for fructose and other sugars.

Over the course of the day, consume a moderate amount of protein: approximately 75 to 100 grams per day. Two eggs contain 13 grams of protein; 4 ounces of chicken breast has 36 grams of protein.

2. **Eat your pound of low-fructose veggies.** Veggies contain lots of fiber and good antioxidants but can also contain fructose. Consume one pound of vegetables per day, or about two cups of vegetables at lunch and at dinner, with an emphasis on vegetables that are low in fructose. Choose vegetables that contain less than 1 gram of fructose per 200-calorie serving, such as artichokes, sauerkraut, spinach, alfalfa sprouts, and peas. Because of the fiber content, vegetables that contain less than 5 grams of fructose (including sweet potatoes, broccoli, squash, and carrots) can also be consumed, as long as you keep your total fructose each day to less than 20 grams.

3. **Forgo alcohol.** In the previous chapters, I outlined the many reasons to take a break from alcohol. In addition to the reasons I've already stated, your favorite cocktail is likely loaded with fructose. Then there's the liver issue. With leptin and the liver so delicately entwined, I implore you to be kind to your liver by eliminating alcohol for the full twenty-one days of the Hormone Reset plan.

4. **Stop snacking.** For my leptin-resistant patients, snacking becomes a habit because they are disconnected from true hunger. You have to break the snacking habit in order to reset your leptin. Eat three meals per day following the guidelines I've described (refer again to the reset guidelines in chapter 2 if necessary, page 41), but don't snack. Time your meals every four to six hours. When leptin is normal—not too high and not too low—you don't feel hungry between meals.

5. **Eat good fats.** Most people, in order to heal their metabolism, need more healthy fat in their diet for optimal health. Good sources include coconut and coconut oil, avocados, butter, nuts, and animal fats (see page 62).

6. **Avoid nightshade fruits and vegetables.** Some people respond
   to nightshade fruits and vegetables with increased inflammation.
   Nightshades contain a chemical named solanine, which may
   interfere with enzymes in your muscles, leading to pain and
   stiffness, and cause digestive problems. You may be exquisitely
   sensitive and may never have realized that nightshades are the
   source of your gut problems and joint discomfort. For three days
   remove all nightshades, including potatoes, tomatoes, eggplant, bell
   peppers, and tomatillos. Avoid American-grown soy, which has been
   hybridized with petunia, a nightshade, to be pesticide resistant.

### SAMPLE MENU

The next page has a suggested menu for resetting your leptin. For
nutritional data, check out the Notes section.[20]

## Supplements

The most proven supplement to help with the damage from fructose
and to reset leptin balance is omega-3s.[21] Remember the polyunsaturated fatty acids (PUFAs) from the Meatless reset? Omega-3s
reverse leptin and insulin resistance, and reduction of leptin levels
by up to 22 percent have been seen with doses of 1,000 milligrams
per day.[22] I suggest 2,000 to 4,000 milligrams per day, and I also
recommend that you discuss the best dose with your practitioner.

## Cell to Soul Practice

Cultivating awareness and gratitude is a major part of the weight
loss strategies that I teach in my integrative medicine practice, yoga
workshops, and online programs. Awareness enables choice and
sustained happiness, and I teach people a long list of ways to break

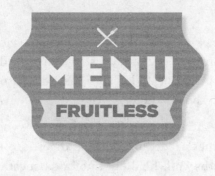

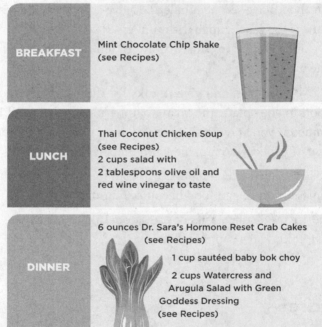

**BREAKFAST**

Mint Chocolate Chip Shake
(see Recipes)

**LUNCH**

Thai Coconut Chicken Soup
(see Recipes)
2 cups salad with
2 tablespoons olive oil and
red wine vinegar to taste

**DINNER**

6 ounces Dr. Sara's Hormone Reset Crab Cakes
(see Recipes)

1 cup sautéed baby bok choy

2 cups Watercress and
Arugula Salad with Green
Goddess Dressing
(see Recipes)

free from the ruts that have developed in their thinking when it comes to food and behavior. I also find that awareness and gratitude are the antidotes to food addiction.

For this reset, I recommend an eating meditation that knits together awareness and gratitude and helps you assimilate the good food you're eating.

Here's how to do it:

1. Before a meal, sit down and turn your complete attention to the food before you. Clear away distractions, like the newspaper or a favorite magazine. (Food addicts tend to also be information addicts—I should know!)

2. Inhale the aroma of your food, which helps your body produce the enzymes needed for optimal digestion. Take three slow, deep breaths while holding your food beneath your nose. Aim for about a five-second inhale and a five-second exhale, without getting too caught up in the numbers. If you're feeling stressed, it can be helpful to pause for five to ten seconds at the top of the inhale.

3. Close your eyes, and give thanks for the hands that got the food to your plate: the farmer (hopefully organic and local, someone you know!), the people who transported the food to you, the folks who provided and prepared it for you.

4. Take your first bite, and put down your fork. Aim to chew thirty times, or until your food becomes liquid.

5. Notice the distinct tastes of your food. Inhale and exhale again before you take your next bite.

## Exercise

Studies show that some women drop their leptin in response to exercise.[23] When you are resetting your leptin pathway, I recommend that you burn calories after dinner. Exercising after dinner allows you to burn extra calories and, ideally, enter a lower energy balance (calories eaten at dinner minus calories burned after dinner) for the all-important, fix-my-leptin overnight fast.

Women are extremely efficient at hanging on to fat at all costs, and I bet that rings true for you. One study showed that overweight men and women respond differently to exercise on a treadmill. Men show no change in their metabolic hormones, and women increase their ghrelin, the hormone that raises appetite.

When your metabolism is slow, exercise does not contribute much to weight loss, as described in the Meatless chapter. You need to sort out your chemistry first and then exercise will be more effective. That's why I suggest less sitting as the first strategy in the Meatless reset. If we look at the role of food versus exercise in helping you lose weight, food takes the lion's share at 75 to 85 percent, and exercise fills in the gap. It is my opinion, based on clinical experience, that once you heal your metabolism, exercise once again plays a more central role in preventing weight regain. Nevertheless, I recommend that you get into the habit of moving your body daily. One of my favorite choices for women is the barre fitness–based form of exercise that blends ballet, pilates, and yoga. The combination lengthens your spine, improves your posture, and boosts your metabolism.

Just remember that vigorous exercise very close to bedtime can interfere with your sleep. At least two hours before bed, go for a brisk walk, practice twenty minutes of yoga, take a quick swim, do five sun salutations, or attend a barre fitness class.

## Test Yourself

If you are curious about where you're starting with leptin, test yourself near the beginning of the Fruitless reset. Additionally, I recommend testing if you have long-standing difficulty with fat loss resistance.

*Fasting leptin.* Ask your doctor to measure your fasting leptin level. An optimal level is between 4 and 6 ng/mL. Above 10 ng/mL is high.

*Reverse T3.* Reverse T3 (reverse triiodothyronine) acts a bit like it's putting your metabolic system in reverse because it blocks the healthy functioning of thyroid hormones T3 and T4. When you eat too much of the wrong foods—usually junk foods, processed foods, and refined carbohydrates—leptin levels rise and your brain sends a signal to the rest of the body to decrease metabolic rate by reducing thyroid hormone production. In other words, leptin resistance slows down your thyroid gland. That means you don't burn fat in your muscles because your basal metabolic rate is lowered. This process, called peripheral (muscle) leptin resistance, explains why some overweight people cannot burn fat with exercise. You are looking for either a high reverse T3 or a low ratio of free T3 to reverse T3. Reverse T3 should be in the lower half of the normal range. For a ratio, simply divide your free T3 by your reverse T3 (using the same units), and the number should be 20 or higher if you're normal. If your ratio is lower than 20, you may have a problem with excess reverse T3.

## Notes from Hormone Resetters

"I am an avid nutrition nut and thought I knew a lot about my body and how to fuel it properly. I was wrong! This [program] taught me so much about myself and has instilled some really beneficial habits that I can benefit from in the long term. I don't recall having lost 12 pounds in less than a month at any time since I hit thirty (I'm forty-four now) so that is impressive to me as well. I would have been happy with 5 pounds so consider this a huge success!"—*Cynthia*

"This has been such an eye-opener in so many ways. The program that Dr. Sara has compiled is so comprehensive, much more than just a simple dietary adjustment that I had initially anticipated.

I've learned so much about how my body functions chemically and organically, what I need and don't need each day. Dr. Sara has presented a wealth of information in order for participants to begin to learn the optimal practices we can each employ daily to live our best lives from soul to cell! I am excited to continue my journey along this path. Although the program is so much greater than the statistics for me, I can share that I lost 14 pounds, dropped roughly 20 points in my fasting blood sugar, and have found a balance for my pH!" —*Jackie*

## Final Word

I'm excited for you to get off fructose, build upon the Meatless and Sugar Free resets, and reset your leptin pathway. We are fixing your hunger switch in this reset. Within seventy-two hours, you will notice more energy, less hunger, dramatically fewer carb cravings, and reduced bloating. You will be well on your way toward less belly fat too! Remember, with each reset, we get closer to figuring out which hormones are standing in the way between you and effortless weight loss. Please pay attention to the messages from your body, and record them in your journal. The details will later prove invaluable as you lose weight and keep it off. Be assured: your Hormone Reset is well underway.

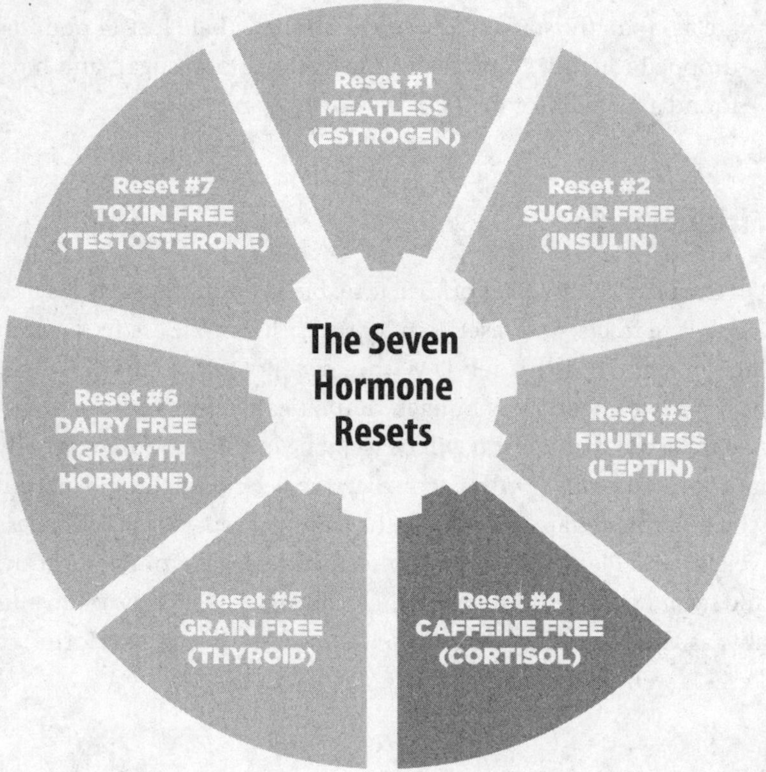

The Seven Hormone Resets

Reset #1
MEATLESS
(ESTROGEN)

Reset #2
SUGAR FREE
(INSULIN)

Reset #3
FRUITLESS
(LEPTIN)

Reset #4
CAFFEINE FREE
(CORTISOL)

Reset #5
GRAIN FREE
(THYROID)

Reset #6
DAIRY FREE
(GROWTH
HORMONE)

Reset #7
TOXIN FREE
(TESTOSTERONE)

# CHAPTER 6

# Caffeine Free

**CORTISOL RESET:** *Days 10 to 12*

It's time to spill the beans. Coffee is our favorite upper, but it's highly addictive and may not be good for you. Ninety percent of Americans drink coffee, and worldwide more than two billion cups of coffee are consumed daily with supply and demand increasing annually. While it may be the most socially acceptable stimulant, many people don't realize it's a drug. What you need to know is that coffee becomes toxic at certain levels and may shift your mood from alert to anxious, disrupt your sleep, and give you palpitations—what I would describe as *overstimulation*. On average, women with sleep problems drink 3.3 cups of caffeinated coffee, tea, or soda daily. Regular consumption of caffeine disconnects you from natural circadian rhythms, which govern your hormonal harmony. Without these natural rhythms, your hormones misfire and you can become fat. That's because coffee elevates cortisol, one of your body's key fat-storage hormones and the ultimate director of your inner world.

When cortisol is too high or too low, it becomes the dark lord of your body. In my experience, when you're highly sensitive to or slow to metabolize it, caffeine leaves you feeling raw and throttled. Living life with chronically high cortisol levels robs you of joy, restful sleep, and control over your weight. Caffeine is another way that women attempt to change their state. Life is hard, and you reach for caffeine to feel less exhausted, or you reach for a bar of chocolate to cope with pain or boredom. I get it, but now it's time to break the vicious cycle of stress, sleeplessness, and fatigue that keeps many of us addicted to caffeine. When you do, you will clearly see how your innocent cup of coffee is keeping you fat. The transformation takes only three days.

## Self-Assessment

How do you know if you are addicted to caffeine and/or need to reset your cortisol? Take the following self-assessment and check off any of the following behaviors or conditions that apply to you now or have occurred in the past six months.

- ☐ Are you one of the 35 million American women who have difficulty sleeping?

- ☐ Do you drink coffee or caffeinated beverages most days of the week?

- ☐ Do you struggle with anxiety or irritability?

- ☐ Do you drink three or more servings of alcohol per week?

- ☐ Do you overeat when stressed?

- ☐ Have you been told you have high and/or low blood sugar? Or is your fasting blood glucose greater than 85 mg/dL?

- ☐ Does the idea of quitting coffee seem outrageous and leave you looking for ways to avoid giving it up?

- ☐ Do you suffer from burnout—physical or emotional exhaustion from chronic stress?

- ☐ Have you been told that your DHEA or testosterone levels are low?

☐ Do you suffer from indigestion, gastroesophageal reflux disease (GERD), or stomach ulcers?

☐ Have you been told you have thinning bones, osteopenia, or osteoporosis?

☐ Do you experience breast tenderness, or has a clinician told you that you have fibrocystic breast change?

☐ Do you have premenstrual syndrome (PMS)?

☐ Do you find, perhaps paradoxically, that the more caffeine you drink, the more tired you feel once the buzz wears off?

### Interpret Your Results

- **If you have five or more of these symptoms,** you are very likely addicted to caffeine and it is robbing you of energy.

- **If you have fewer than five of these symptoms or are unsure,** you might have a caffeine addiction, and I urge you to remove caffeine from your diet periodically, such as once per quarter as outlined in this program.

In my opinion, there are two crucial factors: whether you are genetically hardwired to be slow at metabolizing caffeine (as I am) and what you drink in your coffee (i.e., sugar and/or cream). The takeaway is that I believe you must remove coffee if you want to lose weight, reduce stress, sleep better, live longer, and reset your broken metabolic hormones.

## Tracking Joe

Let's trace the path of your steaming mug of coffee. The caffeine from your cup of joe goes directly from your stomach to your hypothalamus, which regulates hormone levels and prods your pituitary to tell your adrenal glands to release more cortisol. The newly ingested caffeine can also inhibit adenosine, one of your body's natural calming mechanisms. One serving of strong coffee reduces blood flow to your brain by 20 to 30 percent,[1] so you become less resourceful and more irritable.

If you're already stressed, you've got double trouble. Particularly if you are a high-stress type, the elevation in cortisol from the carbs and sugar can raise your blood pressure by constricting your blood vessels.[2]

Increased cortisol may also keep you from sleeping soundly. Cortisol raises blood glucose, which may make you feel foggy, and when it drops, you feel hungry. As your body demands more glucose, the cells say, "*Whoa!* We're shutting down."

The result? You're in a vicious cycle of caffeine, rising cortisol, and unstable blood sugar. Remember insulin resistance? That's when your body doesn't have the capacity to regulate your insulin levels. It turns your waist into a magnet for fat, and because visceral fat has four times the cortisol receptors of fat elsewhere, you keep taking on more fat.

---

### From Dr. Sara's Case Files: Kim, Age Forty-Eight

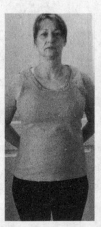
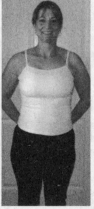

- *Lost 14 pounds, 4 inches off her waist, and 2 inches off her hips.*
- *No longer depressed or feeling bad about how she looks.*
- *"I better understand about my body and hormones and how certain foods can affect how you feel. My hormones are finally back to normal*

*because I feel alive inside. I walk around with a smile on my face now. No more aches and pains in my joints and muscles. Thank you for giving me my life back. I will continue on this journey of great health and better food choices. Food is now my medicine."*

---

## Don't Worry If You're a Coffee Addict

Jill, a patient of mine, felt a true physiological need for caffeine, similar to how a diabetic needs insulin. She couldn't imagine life without coffee. The thought of removing it from her daily routine almost caused her to miss out on one of the most important decisions of her life, which was doing the Hormone Reset Diet. In retrospect, she was glad that she didn't run screaming from my office when I suggested she remove caffeine for twenty-one days. Instead, she dove in and emerged detoxified, caffeine free, and slimmer.

Believe me, I understand. I've been looking high and low for medical reasons to stay addicted to caffeine. But when I put my doctor hat on, I simply have to conclude from the science and the observations in my medical practice that there are strong links between caffeine and weight gain, anxiety, insomnia, and maybe even breast cancer. Over the past decade working with women, and in my own life, I have become a believer in the periodic reset of cortisol with the complete removal of caffeine. I see the proof in my own flat belly and thousands of other flat bellies from the twenty-one-day Hormone Reset Diet. As a recovering caffeine addict, I know your first instinct might be to plead for mercy regarding caffeine and insist on being the exception to the rule. If you stand up to that voice, believe me: you'll be happier, well rested, and thinner!

Never fear. I will make this caffeine free process *painless*, even fun. You'll see the positive results almost immediately, which will give you motivation to keep going. Let's get started!

## ADVICE FOR THE CAFFEINE ADDICT

If you are wigging out about how you can possibly survive without caffeine, I understand. I have an addictive personality. If something is worth doing, it's worth overdoing. When a friend texted me about her favorite new dry shampoo, I found myself applying so much I ran through an entire bottle in one week. When I learned from my friend Dave Asprey that his mycotoxin-free coffee, Bulletproof, was being studied by researchers at Stanford for its effect on cognitive performance, I immediately ordered twenty pounds.

I get it. You need energy, and when there is a strong-smelling, delicious-tasting habit widely available every morning, it's hard to resist. Let me help you with my simple, top-secret strategy to employ in the days leading up to the Big Wean. Ideally, you'll start weaning off caffeine the day you start your Hormone Reset, during Meatless.

- Days 1–3: Say goodbye to your last cup of coffee. Drop your caffeine intake in half.
- Days 3–5: Greet the day with a mug of black tea, no more than two cups.
- Days 6–8: Switch to green or white tea, no more than two cups on days 6 and 7. By day 8, one cup only.
- Day 10: It's herbal tea from now on, baby—for the rest of your Hormone Reset. You've got this!

When you are getting off coffee while living in a coffee-obsessed culture, I urge you to keep your eyes on the prize and on how to create greater ease with weight loss via normalized cortisol.

You may be wondering if you can just switch to decaffeinated coffee. The answer: no. Even though decaf coffee contains smaller amounts of caffeine, like regular coffee it also contains acids that affect blood sugar and cortisol levels, and it has similar effects on cholesterol. Decaf coffee also raises blood pressure and sympathetic nervous system activity.[3]

------

# Women, Stress, Overeating, and Coffee

According to the annual stress survey by the American Psychological Association, women report higher stress than men, are more likely to feel their stress is on the rise, and experience more extreme stress: 25 percent of women state their stress is at an 8 or higher (on a 10-point scale) versus 16 percent of men. Many studies now document what I've seen in my medical office: women are more likely to overeat in response to stress compared with men.[4] Overeating can elevate cortisol, glucose, and insulin levels; fan the fire of persistent inflammation and oxidative stress (which is like the industrial waste of your body and makes you feel prematurely old and toxic); and ultimately, cause weight gain.[5]

Growing evidence suggests that these biological factors work together to accelerate cellular aging by shutting down the telomere care system (the caps on your chromosomes that are an indicator of how fast you are aging).[6] In fact, excess cortisol can shrink the hippocampus by killing brain cells (your hippocampus is where you store memories and regulate emotions). Keep in mind that you're already producing more cortisol as you age. Let's not hasten the process by downing a cup of coffee to rev up.

In my practice, many women have stress stuck in the "redline" position, and stress eating is a typical response, which leads to weight gain. Even worse, chronic stress changes food preferences. Studies show that when you are under stress, you are more likely to eat foods high in sugar or fat, or both. High-fat and sugary foods temporarily comfort your stressed-out brain, and that's why you crave them. But the effects last only while eating, and in the long term, you are left with extra weight and continued cravings.

Chronic stress not only alters your appetite and the types of foods you crave, but it also leads to your losing sleep, drinking more alcohol, and getting less exercise. When you are sleep deprived and hungover, what do you crave? Coffee! All of these factors contribute to weight gain. It started with stress and coffee, and it escalates to overeating the wrong foods and gaining more weight. So, let's keep it simple: dump the caffeine.

Obesity results from chronic problems with energy balance in your body, which is definitely caused in part by high stress. Scientists define stress as the behavioral and physiological responses generated in the face of perceived threat. In girlfriend language, you press the "on" button for your sympathetic nervous system (the fight-or-flight half of your nervous system), which tells your adrenal glands to pump out more adrenaline and cortisol. The system works well for most humans, unless you happen to be female and stuck with a prolonged stressor—such as working at a demanding job, raising a family, or just having a lot on your plate, no pun intended. In this case, you may start to see the ravages of stress and high cortisol: sugar cravings, increased fat storage, and ultimately, stress-induced obesity. Get a group of girlfriends together, and I'm sure you'll hear familiar refrains: *Stressed all the time. Can't lose weight. No time for myself. Can't live without coffee or wine.* It all drives me to drink, but I know better.

You aren't alone. Chronic stress, overeating, and drinking coffee are extremely common and may lead to the type of metabolic harm that sets you up for rapid fat storage and difficulty losing weight. We're again in that vicious cycle of caffeine and cortisol.

## WHY DEEP SLEEP IS GOOD FOR WEIGHT LOSS

*Deep sleep doesn't just feel good. It has solid benefits when it comes to weight loss, and I absolutely love it when I can lose weight during sleep. I advise a few simple rules for great sleep: eat a modest dinner three to four hours before bedtime, turn off screens (TV, tablet, laptop) one hour before bedtime, and refrain from alcohol, which limits deep sleep. (Remember, alcohol also has the unfortunate property of slowing down your fat-burning mechanism.) Most important, become caffeine free so you can fall and stay asleep.*

*Aim for eight hours of sleep. The irony is that caffeine is used to counteract sleepiness, yet consuming caffeine limits your subsequent sleep by disturbing your delicate inner clock. Don't wait to catch up on the weekend—it doesn't work, especially if you're middle aged![7]*

A good night's rest is also good for your waistline. Sleep:

- *increases glucose metabolism and is linked to better blood sugar control;[8]*
- *boosts secretion of growth hormone, which—along with cortisol—regulates belly fat;*
- *activates cellular repair and mends injury;*
- *normalizes cortisol levels during the day (and the corollary: one bad night of sleep raises cortisol);[9] and*
- *improves memory.*

One study showed that women who sleep five hours or less per night weigh more **but eat less** than women who sleep seven hours or more. Clearly, if you want to master your weight, you must master your sleep.

Exercise, relaxation techniques, bedtime rituals—all of these plus the Hormone Reset Diet helps with insomnia. There are countless websites and many books on sleep. One recommended to me that focuses on cognitive behavioral therapy is **Say Good Night to Insomnia** by Gregg D. Jacobs, an insomnia specialist at the Sleep Disorders Center at the University of Massachusetts Memorial Medical Center. Here are a few of his suggestions:[10]

- *Get out of bed within a half hour of the same time each day— even weekends—regardless of how much or little you slept.*
- *Exercise by taking a brisk walk about three or more hours before bedtime, which will improve your sleep by causing a greater rise and fall in your body temperature.*
- *Boost your exposure to morning sun (around ten A.M.) to establish a more consistent circadian rhythm and increase melatonin.*

## About Burnout

Burnout occurs when life demands and chronic stress exceed your coping, which may lead to a state of physical and emotional exhaustion. You may be surprised to learn that emotional eaters *overeat* in response to stress, whereas normal eaters *undereat* in response to stress.[11] Burnout is an important precursor to emotional eating, uncontrolled eating, and weight gain.[12] We know your eating patterns affect whether you gain weight and become obese. Stressed people crave sugar, fat, salt, and alcohol. When your life or work burns you out, there's a much greater likelihood of disordered eating in a misguided attempt to reverse sadness, loneliness, or boredom. In order to reset normal eating, we need to address the root causes of burnout, which can include unrelenting stress, wayward cortisol, fatigue, dependence on coffee, perceived lack of control, and even loss of self-respect.

Let's summarize: When you get stressed, cortisol rises, you overeat, you drink coffee, cortisol rises higher, and then you get fat. Stress makes most women become hypervigilant and struggle with sleep. Coffee, excess cortisol, and even cortisol resistance are the most common hormonal reasons for slow metabolism in women.

## The Science Behind Caffeine Free

We hear all sorts of conflicting information about the benefits and drawbacks of caffeine. You might be wondering just how harmful your cup of coffee is to your health, especially if you're addicted and feeling skeptical about why you need to cut it out of your food plan. I'm here to set the record straight on caffeine and weight, and settle once and for all why you must give up your beloved caffeine for the next three days and for the remainder of your Hormone Resets.

The problem with caffeine is that most people consume too much,

# CAFFEINE: The Scorecard

## PRO

**MAY REDUCE RISK OF:***
- Alzheimer's disease
- Parkinson's
- Stroke
- Liver injury
- Gallstones

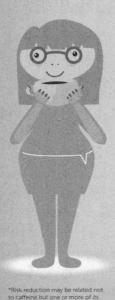

*Risk reduction may be related not to caffeine but one or more of its plant-derived chemicals.

## CON

**MAY MAKE YOU:**
- Jumpy and antsy
- Anxious and irritable
- Sleep worse (affects quality, quantity, how fast you fall asleep, deep sleep)
- Addicted (stimulates dopamine release in the brain, the main chemical mediator of addiction)
- Harms brain development
- Harms your ability to produce GABA, which is Nature's valium
- Engage in other unhealthy behaviors: smoking, excess drinking, and eating red meat

**IMPLICATED IN:**
- Accelerated skin aging
- Fibrocystic breast disease
- Infertility
- PMS
- Osteoporosis
- Hot flashes
- Bruxism (teeth grinding)

**STIMULATES RELEASE OF:**
- Stress neurotransmitters like adrenaline
- Stress hormones like cortisol (may cause "cortisol steal")
- Excess estrogen

**POTENTIAL TOXINS:**
- Acrylamide, a known neurotoxin and probable carcinogen
- Mycotoxins or toxins from mold that may make you fat

**BLOOD SUGAR:**
Triggers high blood sugar, followed by an insulin spike and blood sugar crash, which may prompt weight gain

then show signs of toxicity. How much is too much depends on your age, your cortisol levels, your stress resilience, and how you process caffeine. For the average adult, toxicity occurs at 500 to 1,000 milligrams. Lower doses may cause toxicity if you metabolize caffeine slowly. Furthermore, the cascading hormonal effects from caffeine add to stress and sugar cravings. I know that you coffee worshippers may take offense. Let's start with an objective look at where we are right now with respect to the scientific answer to the question "Cuppa joe—yes or no?" (For citations, go to www.HormoneReset .com/bonus.)

Bottom line? All of us benefit from taking time off from caffeine and seeing what happens—to our sleep, weight, and energy.

### BEYOND COFFEE

We know coffee isn't the only culprit when it comes to our nation's amped-up stress boosters. You can suffer from caffeine toxicity in many ways. We drive ourselves hard and expect our bodies to meet every demand we heap upon them. But sometimes this backfires, particularly when you reach a certain threshold of caffeine. Furthermore, your safe level of caffeine and your liver's ability to detoxify you from caffeine declines with age and with liver congestion. Your cortisol levels naturally rise with age; a person of sixty-five has far higher levels of circulating cortisol than a twenty-five-year-old, and drinking caffeine may contribute to menopausal weight gain.

When you drink too much caffeine, you're robbing your own bank. The theft results from the high biological cost of overstimulation, excess production of stress hormones, and ultimately, depleted reserves of your adrenal glands. When you're overweight and stressed, the scorecard favors periodic removal of caffeine.

## Caffeine Free: The Three-Day Reset for Cortisol

It's time to stop robbing your body's bank: eliminate caffeine and reset cortisol immediately. Try it for the remainder of the twenty-one days. You might like how you feel so much that you continue, and I strongly urge you to do so.

## CAFFEINE FREE RULES: DO THESE EACH DAY

Follow these simple yet powerful rules to reset your stress and cortisol levels, and remember to continue the rules you've already implemented from the previous resets:

1. **Eliminate all caffeine.** This includes coffee, black tea, green tea, soda, and energy drinks.
   *Caffeine Alternatives List:* Hot water with lemon and cayenne, hot water with cardamom, herbal teas, mushroom teas (see Resources).

2. **Continue eating one pound of vegetables per day,** along with healthy, plant-based fats and proteins and small servings of low-glycemic fruits.

3. **Keep your net carbs between 20 and 49 grams per day.**

### CAFFEINE AMOUNTS

*When you're overweight and highly sensitive to caffeine and cortisol, it doesn't matter if you have two cups or ten cups of caffeine; the drawbacks are similar.*

- *A typical 8-ounce (240-milliliter) cup of instant coffee contains about 100 milligrams of caffeine—about twice as much as a cup of tea or a 12-ounce (360-milliliter) can or bottle of soda.*

- *One ounce of dark chocolate contains 12 milligrams of caffeine, which is why I suggest that you eat no more than one ounce of dark chocolate (80 percent cacao or higher) but skip the coffee.*

## SAMPLE MENU

Here is a suggested menu for resetting your cortisol. For nutritional data, check out the Notes section.[13]

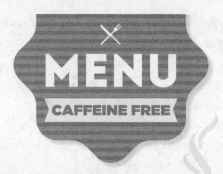

**BREAKFAST**

1 cup hot water with lemon and cayenne (no caffeine)

2 Protein Egg Muffins (see Recipes)

**LUNCH**

Detox shake such as Dr. Sara's Basic Vanilla or Chocolate Shake (see Recipes), with 1 cup spinach and 1 tablespoon MCT oil

**DINNER**

6 ounces Ground Turkey Endive Roll-Ups (see Recipes)

1 cup Creamy Goddess Greens Soup (see Recipes)

1 cup steamed cauliflower

2 cups Kale and Beet Salad (see Recipes) with oil and vinegar or lemon

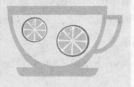

1 Dr. Sara's Hormone Reset Brownie (see Recipes)

## STAY OFF THE SAUCE

When you remove your upper, you won't need your downer—
otherwise known as alcohol. But as a woman of a certain age, I need
a periodic reminder of why it's not a good idea to pour a glass of wine
at six P.M.

Alcohol raises your cortisol level and makes you more stressed,
not less. Sure, there's the little buzz at the beginning, and who doesn't
love that? But it's another hijacker of the restorative sleep you need to
clean up the metabolic mess that you're in. It also raises breast cancer
risk, even at low doses of as little as three glasses of zin per week.

You will not be surprised to learn that alcoholics have a problem
with the stress-response loop in their bodies, particularly in the
hippocampus, the part of the brain where you perform memory
organization and consolidation, plus emotional regulation.[14] Not
only does the brain shrink and stop rewiring, but also, when you
drink more than two servings per day, 639 genes are changed for
the worse. Why should you care about the 639 genes? They regulate
vitally important functions, such as the actions of the cortisol
receptor (known more generally as the glucocorticoid receptor),
mineral transport (such as zinc, performed by the SLC39A10 gene),
and inflammation (IL1R1).

The bottom line: keep your fat loss going by resetting your cortisol,
and stay off alcohol through the full twenty-one days of your Hormone
Reset. If you need some concrete ways to help you, see Ways to Wean
Yourself Off Alcohol in chapter 3 (page 65).

## SIX WAYS TO HELP YOU WAKE UP IN THE MORNING

1. **ChiWalking.** Lose weight, strengthen your core, and improve
   your posture—all before breakfast! Check out the Exercise
   section (page 141) for instructions.

2. **Sun salutations.** There's no better way to wake up than saluting the sun! Go to a beginner's yoga class or follow the instructions on my YouTube channel.

3. **Bellows breathing.** This energizing yogic breathing is better than any upper. Inhale and exhale fast through your nose, with your mouth shut. Aim for one to three breath cycles per second, and continue for ten to thirty seconds. Your breath duration in and out should be equivalent, but as short as possible, like a bellows. Don't be afraid to make some noise.

4. **Meditation.** News flash! Meditation isn't the same as sleeping or just some woo-woo way to focus the mind. On the contrary, a short meditation can leave you feeling energized and alert, and it's a killer swap for caffeine. Find a comfortable cross-legged position and take a few deep breaths. Then slowly start to breathe normally. When thoughts arise, simply bring your awareness back to your breath.

5. **Five minutes of burst training.** You don't need anything fancy to get your morning blood flowing. Do twenty-five push-ups, really taking time with the "down" part of the push-up, and practice staying present with what you see while you get your heart moving.

6. **Five minutes of fun-factor cardio.** There's no excuse not to do five minutes of fun cardio at home. Blast some Taylor Swift, run up and down the stairs, anything that gets you a little sweaty will do. Just don't overdo it.

## Supplements

When it comes to your caffeine-free reset, I recommend supplements that increase your metabolic rate safely without overstimulating your nervous system, a side effect I often observe with weight-reduction formulas that contain caffeine. One of my favorite supplements is decaffeinated green tea extract. Here's why: your risk versus benefit from caffeine is subject to your own individual tolerance, and that's why I believe everybody benefits from taking time off from caffeine and seeing what happens with sleep and weight loss. Green tea clearly has benefits for the majority of people based on the best evidence, but be aware that much of the health improvements with regard to weight loss and insulin sensitivity seems to result from polyphenols—a group of powerful antioxidants from tea leaves— not necessarily from caffeine.[15] Green tea (*Camellia sinensis*) contains the highest concentration of polyphenols, called catechins.[16] The most abundant is epigallocatechin-3-gallate (EGCG), which is linked to cancer-prevention activity,[17] lower blood glucose,[18] reduced risk of heart disease,[19] and modest weight loss of up to 8 pounds.[20] I recommend EGCG at a dose of 400 milligrams twice per day. You get the benefit without the caffeine.

## Cell to Soul Practice

In my cell-to-soul philosophy, which is informed by Chinese medicine, Tibetan medicine, and ayurveda, the urge for caffeine is an important sign that the body, mind, and/or spirit are out of balance. I've learned to get curious about cravings and query the deeper message coming from our bodies. You might be burned out, need more social connection and love, need more sleep, or discover that you may not like your work or your spouse. Whatever you learn, you are much more likely to find a source of true energy within yourself that doesn't deplete your body. You might try a restorative yoga pose like butterfly, a green smoothie, a cup of hot water with fresh lemon and cayenne, a good conversation with a girlfriend, or even an adaptogenic supplement that balances the body. Sources of true energy provide a more modulated ride that doesn't have extreme highs and lows, and the result is more-stable blood sugar, fewer sugar cravings, and no more hormonal roller-coaster rides.

I often look to other cultures to see their perspective on stimulants like coffee. In ayurveda, the five-thousand-year-old Indian system of natural healing and traditional medicine, coffee overactivates your mind and takes you further from the goal of balance, which should be felt as the stilling of the mind. Ayurveda translates as the science of life, and at the root of balanced living is optimal digestion of not just physical nutrients but emotional and spiritual food as well. When you are in a state of balance, your nervous system and endocrine system perform well without stimulants and your energy is consistent. No roller coaster. Just a sustained, buoyant feeling of energy and optimism, and it rests on the key circadian driver of deep sleep each night. This is called the *sattva*, the ideal state of calm and equilibrium.

In Chinese medicine, you are born with a fixed amount of energy, known as prenatal chi, which you received from your parents. Your prenatal chi cannot be supplemented; it can only be conserved. Coffee depletes your natal chi. Because of the difficulty of giving up coffee and the importance of resetting cortisol, I recommend "left nostril breathing," which my friend and Harvard psychologist Sharon Melnick calls "back-to-sleep" breathing.

## Left Nostril Breathing (or Back-to-Sleep Breathing)

Coffee makes you more reactive, meaning that you're less able to hit the pause button before you react to some emotional trigger. Besides the weight loss you can expect when you quit coffee, another benefit is that you can more easily shift from being reactive to being proactive, which is a cardinal sign of stress resilience, emotional growth, and psychological maturity.

Being reactive is good for grim conditions, such as hunting wild animals for sustenance or self-defense. But it's not good for enduring relationships, a happy marriage, satisfying parenting, personal growth, quality of life, or—for our purposes—achieving and maintaining lean body mass. As my colleague Rick Hanson taught me, reactivity makes us "overlearn from bad experiences and underlearn from good ones": we're Teflon for positive experiences and Velcro for negative ones. Being reactive, or triggered emotionally like a cornered animal, feels bad and sidelines your ability to tap into more advanced emotional resources. It leads to overeating, drinking too much alcohol, watching too much TV, maybe even using shopping as a balm. Most of all, reactivity limits your body's repair mechanisms, which are essential to keeping you in physical and emotional balance.

Left nostril breathing can help you get a handle on your reactivity. Do it when you wake up too early or are in a potentially explosive situation.

Here's how to do it:

- Cover your right nostril with your right thumb, and inhale through your left nostril while counting slowly to ten.

- Hold your breath for another count of ten.

- Move your right ring finger to cover your left nostril, release your thumb to uncover your right nostril, and exhale through your right nostril while slowly counting to ten.

- Inhale through your right nostril while counting slowly to ten.

- Hold your breath for another count of ten.

- Move your thumb back to cover your right nostril and exhale through your left nostril while slowly counting to ten.

- Repeat this sequence three times.

## Exercise

When you are resetting your cortisol pathway, you need to perform "adaptive" exercise so that you don't raise your cortisol even further and fry your hardworking adrenal glands. As you know by now, cortisol is produced in your adrenals. When you run around with stress overload, certain forms of exercise, particularly running and spinning, raise cortisol. I recommend ChiWalking or jogging instead. The benefit to ChiWalking or running compared with the regular way that you walk or run is twofold: you retain more energy and prevent injury. I'm a runner. In my twenties and thirties, I experienced several knee injuries, including a constantly tight IT (iliotibial) band. At some point, I felt like the impact might be too much on my poor body, and I began to look for ways to avoid further stress. ChiWalking is a great choice if you find walking stale or if walking doesn't seem to help with losing weight.

Danny and Katherine Dreyer get the credit for knitting together the concepts of tai chi with walking, jogging, and running in their book *ChiWalking*. However, I have to credit my dad for my interest too, because I remember seeing a *ChiRunning* book (also by Danny and Katherine Dreyer) in his study while I was home from college. ChiWalking is different from regular walking because you use your body more efficiently and reduce impact. The magic is in the engagement of your core muscles and the change in the foot strike.[21]

Here's a primer on how to do it:

1. Place your feet together, distributing your weight evenly. Wiggle your toes, gently bend your knees, and imagine a triangle of your weight spread evenly between your big toe, little toe, and heel.

2. Align your spine. Put your hand on your heart and lengthen through your crown, to reduce swayback (common for women, which causes low back pain).

3. Keep your chin level with the ground. Look to the horizon, and allow the information that comes in through your eyes to energize you. Relax your eye muscles, and relax your body.

4. Relax your shoulders. Your shoulders are not earrings—they do not belong up near your head, in the vicinity of your earlobes. Let your arms swing from your shoulders, back and forth, like you're rubbing a volleyball in front of you at belly level.

5. Engage your *dan tien*. Yes, I know it's a weird, new term, but just focus on this: your *dan tien* is where your life force is centered. It's in an important place: three fingerbreadths below your navel and two inches deep into your core. Pull your energy into your body, concentrating at that spot, and focus it.

6. Place all your weight onto one leg (this leg becomes your yang). Lift the foot of your other leg, which is now empty of weight (this leg becomes your yin), and move your foot forward to take a natural step. Transfer your weight from your front foot to your back foot, until all your weight is on the back foot. Lift the toes of your front foot and turn it on your heel until the toes point outward at a 45-degree angle, then place your front foot back on the floor and shift weight to your front foot. Pick up your back foot and move it toward your front foot. You are now ChiWalking, sister!

7. Lean forward at the ankles to walk faster.

### AFTER THREE DAYS: WHAT'S NEXT?

*After you complete your three days of resetting cortisol by going caffeine free, it's time to focus on the bigger project of resetting your inner clock to lock in your improved metabolism. Studies show the connection between an inner clock gone haywire and getting fat.[22] What's the best way to reset your inner clock?*

- *Get at least twenty minutes of bright sunlight each morning. This helps you make more melatonin, which is another inner clock regulator, along with cortisol.*

- *Make bedtime darker by removing from your bedroom all exterior light, alarm clocks, toys, and other electronics with LED lights. The light suppresses your pineal gland (the endocrine gland in the middle of your brain that secretes melatonin).*

- *Take your vitamins. Melatonin is made in your body from serotonin, and you can make more with the help of a little vitamin B6 and vitamin C. Aim for 50 to 100 milligrams per day of vitamin B6 and 1,000 to 2,000 milligrams per day of vitamin C.*

- *Actively hit the "pause" button on stress by making it a habit every day to feel and express gratitude or any other positive emotion. I have a favorite app on my iPhone called Inner Balance that helps me do this, or I share a long, lingering hug with someone I love. We know that hugs raise oxytocin, the hormone of love, bonding, and social connection, and it's your best ally against chronic stress.*

*After you complete the seventy-two-hour Caffeine Free reset, I urge you to stay off caffeine for the rest of the twenty-one-day Hormone Reset. Many of my clients find that weight loss and maintenance are easier without the battery acid.*

———————

## Test Yourself

There are two tests that I recommend in the Caffeine Free reset: heart rate variability and diurnal cortisol.

*Heart rate variability (HRV),* which is at the core of research conducted by the Institute of HeartMath, is a measure of the naturally occurring beat-to-beat changes in heart rate/heart rhythms. It serves as a critical method for gauging human health and stress resiliency. You can measure HRV with your iPhone (using the app I just mentioned, GPS for the Soul, which can be downloaded for free, or Inner Balance, which requires a sensor for your ear-lobe to measure your HRV) or use HeartMath's handheld heart monitor, the emWave. HeartMath methodology is based on the fact that the time between each beat of your heart varies according to emotional arousal. Loss of variability is a sign of inner emotional stress and waning adaptive suppleness, as well as of possible heart disease.

*Diurnal cortisol.* We produce different amounts of cortisol at different points throughout the day; ideally, it's a gentle downward slope with the highest amount produced in the morning and then a slowly decreasing amount because that sets up the best circadian rhythm for energy during the day and sleep at night. While you can get a single blood test in the morning to test your cortisol, the diurnal test is quite useful because it indicates your cortisol level at four points throughout the day, between six A.M. and ten P.M., rather than basing your findings on one snapshot. (You can test your cortisol levels yourself using the labs listed in Resources.) With more information on the pattern of your cortisol levels, you'll know the best option for treatment—i.e., if your cortisol is too high at night, you need methods to wind down and lower your cortisol, and if your cortisol is too low in the morning, you may need to do more stimulating exercise, such as jogging or a dance class.

## Notes from Hormone Resetters

"I used to enjoy swimming and I haven't done it in over a year. For some reason I gravitated back to it this week. . . . It's like natural caffeine. Nothing wakes you up like jumping into a cold pool! It also just feels very meditative, nurturing, and gentle on my body." —*Holly*

"I have been ignoring my coworkers' resistance to my giving up coffee. We're a coffee-fueled org, and I think my choice is a threat to some folks. I just keep saying, 'It feels right for me right now. I'm not sure what I'll do long-term.' Sticking to my guns!" —*Ashley*

"I wasn't too excited to get rid of my coffee and wine . . . but wow, I've learned so much and feel good. And the bonus: losing 20 pounds. Yup, 20!" —*Renee*

"I am off caffeine and sleeping better, waking up feeling rested without that feeling of 'I need coffee.' This REAL energy is so much better than any caffeine fix! I have not had any sugar and don't even want it! I am working on no snacking between meals, which has been kind of hard since I don't really eat large meals when I do eat. I have lost several pounds, and I just feel happy inside!" —*Vivian*

## Final Word

I have found that feeling chronically stressed is one of the greatest obstacles to weight loss. Yet most of my patients feel chronically stressed. No wonder they have trouble losing weight! Learning how to de-stress is crucial to reaching your weight-loss goals and being able to dump the caffeine.

Stress is in the eye of the beholder. You might think stress is based on external factors, but it's your internal response to the external stressors that matters most. The good news is that this inside job creates an exciting opportunity to navigate your response to external factors—that is, your internal landscape is under your control.

I know a woman who has learned a mantra from a teacher informed by Christian and Eastern traditions: *I give up my desire for esteem and affection, for power and control, for security and survival.*

Now, *that's* letting go of the need to react to your emotional buttons.

We all have stressors we can't control. But you are creating the emotional distress that accompanies chronic stress. Women are wired to take on others' needs. But I want you to focus on actively de-stressing by not just getting off caffeine but also owning your role in stress, establishing boundaries on what you can reasonably accomplish within your current bandwidth, and applying proven strategies to improve your sleep and reduce your stress load. Detoxifying your food and drink won't have the full impact if you continue to keep your mind and spirit toxic with your thoughts and emotions. We all need to address the mental, emotional, and psychological toxins in addition to meat, sugar, and caffeine. Getting off coffee is a big step, but you also need to make a point each day to de-stress and reset your cortisol levels. Your body will reward you by repairing your metabolism and losing stubborn fat. I can feel your commitment! And if that commitment wanes, act "as if" and I promise it will become a habit. Amen!

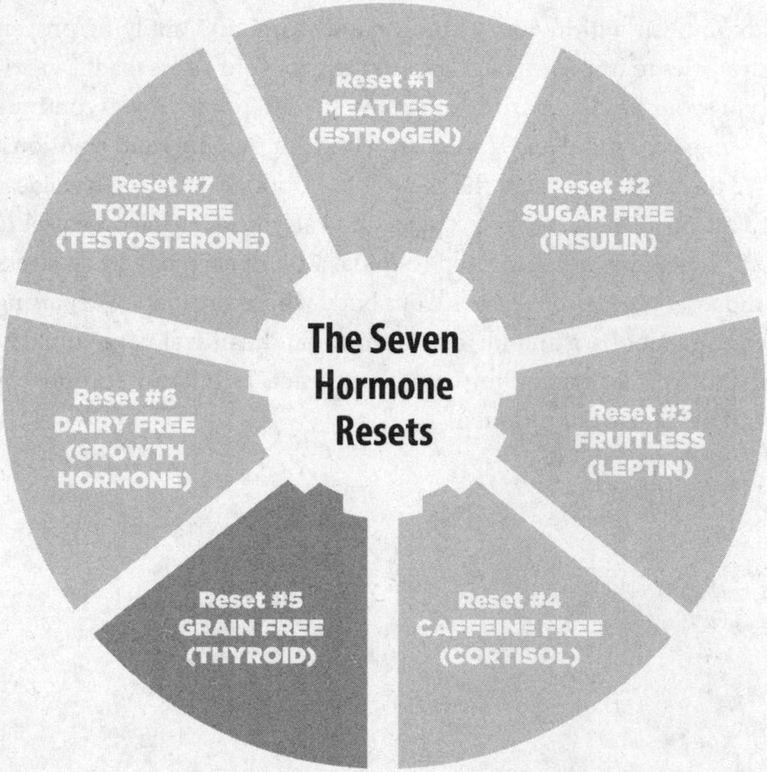

The Seven Hormone Resets

Reset #1
MEATLESS
(ESTROGEN)

Reset #2
SUGAR FREE
(INSULIN)

Reset #3
FRUITLESS
(LEPTIN)

Reset #4
CAFFEINE FREE
(CORTISOL)

Reset #5
GRAIN FREE
(THYROID)

Reset #6
DAIRY FREE
(GROWTH
HORMONE)

Reset #7
TOXIN FREE
(TESTOSTERONE)

## CHAPTER 7

# Grain Free

**THYROID RESET: *Days 13 to 15***

I have an important announcement to make, so kindly pay attention. *Nearly every person who struggles with weight has an issue with grains, particularly those that contain gluten.* When your goal is getting lean, eating grains is like throwing gas on a fire; it's an explosive combination that may thwart your weight-loss goals.

Most grains have a fairly high-glycemic index, meaning that after one to two hours, your blood sugar surges. Unfortunately, foods that spike your blood sugar are chemically addictive. They spur inflammation in your body and keep you in a downward spiral of craving and a growing waistline. Grains are low in nutrient density compared with plants or animals. Grains do more than make you fat: there's a newly discovered link between grains and your hormone levels of leptin, thyroid, and insulin. So, what to do? My recommendation is to remove grains and delight in the effects over the three-day Grain Free reset.

## Self-Assessment

If life without bread seems like a life not worth living, take a deep breath. Your first step is to complete the following self-assessment to determine the extent of your grain-related issues. Do you have or have you experienced in the past six months . . .

☐ Recurring abdominal bloating and/or pain? Frequent or smelly gas? Food poisoning? (Food poisoning puts you at greater risk of problems with gluten.) Constipation or diarrhea? Diagnosis of irritable bowel disease or acid reflux (GERD)?

☐ A first- or second-degree relative with celiac disease?

☐ Anxiety, depression, and/or schizophrenia?

☐ Migraines or other headaches?

☐ Unexplained weight gain? Difficulty losing weight?

☐ Short stature? As a child, did you have low birth weight (i.e., less than 5 pounds)? Attention deficit? Autism?

☐ Joint pain or aches? Bone pain?

☐ Brain fog? Chronic fatigue?

☐ Hair loss? Chronic eczema or acne? Unexplained skin rashes?

☐ Vitamin and/or mineral deficiencies? Iron-deficient anemia?

☐ Unexplained infertility? Menstrual disorders? Repeated miscarriages (three or more)?

☐ A loss of balance and coordination? Difficulty walking or walking with a wide gait?

☐ Restless legs syndrome?

☐ Thyroid antibodies, also known as autoimmune thyroiditis or Hashimoto's disease, or another autoimmune condition?

### Interpret Your Results

- **If you have five or more of these symptoms,** you very likely have a problem with grains, particularly gluten. You have the hallmark symptoms that show inflammatory, allergic, digestive, autoimmune, mood, or cognitive problems. Go grain free and consider asking your doctor for a blood (serum) test of your response to gluten (see the Test Yourself section, page 169).

- **If you have fewer than five of these symptoms or are unsure,** you might have a problem with grains, and I urge you to perform the three-day Grain Free reset.

---

### Meet Gena

---

*Gena Lee Nolin, a star of the 1990s hit TV series Baywatch, seemed like the picture of perfect health at forty-one. With bronze skin, shining eyes, and a killer bod, she was the woman we all wanted to be. But internally she suffered.*

*Over a short period of time, she developed a baffling array of symptoms: exhaustion, brain fog, bloating, depression, and hair loss. When she got pregnant, her symptoms worsened. Soon, she developed a life-threatening heart condition (due to a thyroid issue that was misdiagnosed), which required medications with many serious side effects. And then there was the weight she simply couldn't lose. After each of her pregnancies, it took Herculean efforts to fit into her skimpy red bathing suit. Gena ate perfectly and exercised hard with a trainer nearly every day—and her weight would barely budge.*

*Like millions of American women, Gena was struggling with undiagnosed thyroid disease. Thyroid problems leave women feeling anything but beautiful. After they describe their debilitating symptoms, they often find themselves stigmatized by friends, family, and doctors, and they blame themselves for not being able to get their act together. Gena was finally diagnosed by one astute doctor as having autoimmune thyroiditis, a disease in which the thyroid gland is attacked by the body's own cells. Approximately 90 percent of Americans with low thyroid function have autoimmune thyroiditis, which means that one in every one thousand people are affected. But many people have experiences similar to Gena's; it took ten years for her to get the cor-*

rect diagnosis, and she was told more than fifty times by doctors that there was nothing wrong. Gena isn't alone.

After finally receiving the correct diagnosis in 2009, Gena went on an aggressive campaign to heal her body. She kicked grains to the curb and has been gluten free for more than three years. She began thyroid medication. And within seventy-two hours, Gena was a new woman. "I was almost symptom free," she told me in amazement. When she fixed her low thyroid function through cutting out grains and augmenting her thyroid hormone levels, Gena lost weight and felt great, and life became a walk on the beach—and she published a superb book about it, called Beautiful Inside and Out: Conquering Thyroid Disease with a Healthy, Happy, "Thyroid Sexy" Life.[1] I was so inspired by Gena's powerful story and her happy ending, I even wrote the foreword to her book!

Check out Gena's awesome website, www.officialgenaleenolin .com, where she answers questions and offers an authentic conversation between women around the world, and conference calls with top doctors. Gena truly found the grace of hormonal reset and is applying her newfound vitality to spread the word!

## The Science Behind Grain Free

It's important to recognize why both gluten and grains can be bad for your gut—and your weight-loss efforts. Gluten is a protein found in some grains, but not all. If you love your carbs, there are plenty of healthy nongrain alternatives, such as sweet potatoes, yams, and plantains.

Grains are like the bully on the playground, pretending to be your friend but eventually causing you to be miserable instead. I should know: when I went grain free several years ago, I flipped the switch on fat storage and lost weight. Here are the top ten scary facts about grains:

1. Grains can keep you addicted to the very foods that are causing the worst damage by making you hungry for more. Under
these conditions, it's no wonder you are having problems losing weight.

2. Grains (yes, even gluten-free ones) cause blood sugar spikes
that lead to your body depositing more fat, usually at your
waist. These carbs enter your bloodstream too quickly, in the
form of glucose, causing your blood sugar to spike, followed
by an insulin surge, which leads to biological addiction. This
is the pattern that is linked not just to getting fat but also to
the development of diabetes and even Alzheimer's disease.[2]
Grains, bread, and potatoes are the most positively correlated
foods when it comes to how much a food raises your blood
sugar.[3]

3. In one study of 117,366 men and women aged forty to seventy-
four, eating more refined grains predicted an 80 percent
increased risk of heart disease.[4] In the United States, 80 percent of grains are consumed in the form of refined flour.

4. Men and women respond differently to refined grains when
it comes to metabolic syndrome (the constellation of symptoms that signal a broken metabolism, including a thick waist,
abnormal cholesterol, high blood pressure, and/or problems
with blood glucose). Men are at greater risk for metabolic
syndrome when they eat a higher proportion of carbohydrates
in their diet, but women are at risk for metabolic syndrome
based solely on their intake of refined grains, including rice
and pasta.

5. More carbs may reduce your fertility, even if you're otherwise a
healthy woman.[5] The worst offenders are high-glycemic-index
foods, such as cold breakfast cereals, white rice, and potatoes.

6. In a Harvard study of eighty-three thousand women, an intake
combination of lower carbohydrates, higher proteins, and

higher fats was not linked to risk of heart disease; in fact, vegetable sources of fat and protein were tied to a moderately reduced risk. A higher glycemic load in the same study was associated with a 90 percent greater risk of heart disease.[6]

7. Refined grains are linked to weight gain in women.[7] Examples include white rice, pasta, pastries, doughnuts, and anything with white flour, including cookies and cake.

8. Twenty years ago, we were told to eat more grains and cut the fat. Since then, the diagnosis of diabetes has tripled, according to the Centers for Disease Control and Prevention.[8]

9. Toxins from mold, called mycotoxins, are found in wheat and other grains. They make you fat and cranky. In one study, 65 percent of cereals contained at least one mycotoxin.[9]

10. Grains contain potentially harmful anti-nutrients beyond gluten, including

   • Agglutinins, a type of lectin that may cause leaky gut, dysbiosis (overgrowth of bad bacteria in the gut), and inflammation;

   • Phytates (or phytic acid) that can cause leaky gut and reduce the absorption of certain minerals (calcium, iron, magnesium, potassium, and zinc), which may lead to mineral deficiency; and

   • Digestive enzyme inhibitors, which may cause leaky gut and dysbiosis and stimulate the immune system (also found in dairy, legumes, nuts, and seeds).

   The solution to these dire facts? Go grain free! See how you feel when you cut out the grains in the next step of your food rehab.

## Modified Paleo

How could it be that modern grains are linked to blood sugar problems and getting fat? It turns out that the grains common in the

Standard American Diet (SAD) came into the picture for humans relatively recently. Long before grains, we ate vegetables, seeds, nuts, and wild game. Our Paleolithic ancestors were adapted to a diet high in fiber, clean (and anti-inflammatory) proteins, and phytonutrients. So, it makes sense that many of us haven't adapted to eating grains.

That's where the Paleo diet comes in. This diet is supposed to mimic the food of our cavewoman ancestors. It includes fresh fruits and vegetables, meat, and seafood, while eliminating whole grains. Its stance on grains? That they don't provide adequate nutritional support, and our bodies weren't designed to digest them. Paleo makes a lot of sense to me, but I highly recommend some modifications for women. Although I agree with the consensus to cut out the grains, women must be careful with carb restriction. Cutting out all carbs on a very low carb or ketogenic diet may lead to thyroid problems, mood issues, adrenal dysfunction, and heart complications. For that reason, I designed the Hormone Reset Diet to eliminate the grains but not cut your carbs so low that you're bingeing or otherwise having your best intentions backfire.

Overall, the Paleo diet helps most men and some women get lean. So, let me share the important tweaks proven to make Paleo work for you.[10]

- If you're trying to lose weight, focus on your pound per day of vegetables and you'll get the carbs you need.

- Eat carbs, such as the beloved roasted sweet potato, at night twice per week.

- Make sure to get your vitamin D,[11] because most of us are deficient and it boosts metabolism. The Paleo diet works a whole lot better with sunlight (to improve your circadian rhythm) and added vitamin D—I recommend 2,000 IU (international units) per day.

## YOUR TASTE BUDS ARE TURNING OVER

*I want to honor you for all the effort you've put into your Hormone Reset up to this point, and you're more than halfway there! The good news is that it gets easier starting now, and one reason is that you are losing your taste for the foods that harm your metabolism. Here are a few startling and hopeful facts about your taste buds, which is where you sense the nutrients that you eat:*[12]

- *You rebuild new taste buds once every two weeks, so after going grain free you will have a whole new set!*

- *Your taste buds use receptors for the following tastes: salty, sour, bitter, sweet, and umami. (If "umami" is a new word, keep in mind that the Japanese define it as a "pleasant savory taste" that is distinct from "salty.")*

- *Each taste bud contains approximately fifty to one hundred taste cells.*

- *You have three thousand to ten thousand taste buds in your mouth, on the tongue, palate, and esophagus.*

- *Many women are in the habit of eating sweet foods. Because your taste buds are reset every two weeks, you will find that the foods that serve you best will start to taste better. You may notice during the Grain Free reset that steamed broccoli and spinach taste yummier than they did on Day 1.*

- *Advances from genomic medicine have taught us that much of taste is genetically determined. For instance, you may inherit the taste of increased bitterness from a parent (the gene is called TAS2R38), and every time you eat cruciferous vegetables, such as broccoli or cabbage or Brussels sprouts, or some other foods, including soy products and dark chocolate, you find they taste bitter and you do not enjoy these foods. Never fear! We have many other less bitter, nonstarchy vegetables for you to choose from, including asparagus, bell pepper, carrots, squash, and zucchini.*

-------

# The Truth About Gluten

We can't have a conversation about grains without talking about gluten, which is in so many of our favorite products. The word "gluten" is actually the Latin word for "glue"; it is the protein found in wheat, barley, and rye that provides elasticity to baked goods, such as bread, cereal, and pizza.

The problem is that gluten may make you fat. When ingested, gluten can sound an alarm in your gut and brain, trigger immune overreaction, increase appetite, and hook you into overeating. It can punch holes in the wall of the gut lining, leading to bloating, creating an aching belly, and causing your immune system to malfunction.

Even a small amount can cause discomfort. After staying off gluten and losing weight, I tried one slice of bread. Immediately I became bloated and couldn't zip my cute jeans.

While gluten is widely consumed in the Western world, here's the rub: it turns out that gluten is quite difficult to digest for the majority of people. You need special enzymes to break it down. Some experts believe that up to 80 percent of the population lacks sufficient enzymes needed to break down and assimilate gluten. It's like trying to eat a whole onion—it's a lot easier to consume when you chop the onion into smaller pieces, the way enzymes chop your gluten into smaller pieces that your body can handle more efficiently. When the gluten proteins are not sufficiently chopped down to size, they permeate the underlying immune tissue of the gut and lead to overstimulation of the immune system. That means your immune system can backfire and actually make you sick, such as with autoimmune conditions like Hashimoto's disease.

In fact, several of the most serious health conditions we face, including diabetes, thyroid disease, and even autism (plus about fifty-two other diseases), may be linked to gluten consumption. The consensus among scientists is that gluten-containing grains are a *mistake of evolution*—that is, gluten creates a perfect storm of the conditions needed for human disease.[13]

When you eat refined carbohydrates, gluten causes blood sugar to spike. People who go on a gluten-free diet are thereby avoiding the refined wheat products that cause their blood sugar to spike and then drop, which may account for the health benefits experienced by those who go gluten free.[14]

I'm in awe when I consider how much work our gut does for us, and often without the appreciation and understanding that it rightfully deserves. Did you know that 60 percent of your immune system is directly below a single layer of cells in your small intestine (that's the connector between your stomach and large intestine)? That single layer of cells protecting us from the outside world makes us quite vulnerable. It's the true reason that gluten wrecks the gut so easily. Imagine if the windows of your home were made of aluminum foil instead of sturdy glass. During a storm, you'd feel pretty insecure. Over time, your "window" would probably start looking pretty haggard. The rain, wind, and cold air would inevitably start to come in. It's the same with your gut. You need to take good care of it and protect it from the elements, and you will be much safer in the long run.

Unfortunately, gluten is ubiquitous. Look no further than your local café counter, which glistens with moist pastries, mouthwatering muffins, and bready breakfast sandwiches. These treats may seem like a reward for your hard work, but for some of us they are really the booby prize. You'll find gluten in many prepared products too. It isn't found only in processed foods but in cosmetics and household products as well.[15]

Gluten has become the dietary villain of the decade, and the backlash has led to an astounding growth of gluten-free breads, muffins, and desserts—all of which I consider to be gluten-free junk food. In fact, the market for gluten-free foods is a $6.3 billion industry and growing, up 33 percent since 2009.[16] Companies are touting their gluten-free products, even when they never had any gluten to begin with! The practice has become so widespread that Trader Joe's poked fun at it by offering gluten-free greeting cards.

# The Gluten Sensitivity Spectrum

The experts agree that there is a spectrum of problems with gluten ranging from no symptoms at one extreme to full-blown celiac disease at the other extreme. (Celiac disease is an autoimmune reaction to gluten in genetically predisposed individuals whereby ingestion of gluten damages the small intestine.) Many of us may exist in the gray area in between, with mild to moderate and sometimes vague symptoms, including increased appetite and the dreaded "wheat belly," the increase in fat around your belly (see Wheat Belly: A Balanced Look, page 160).

What I've observed over the past two decades is that most people seem to be sensitive to gluten; it's simply a matter of when this sensitivity rears its ugly head. It's time to free yourself from the tyranny of gluten. I highly encourage you to choose health by eliminating gluten from your diet. If you have a hunch that you might be sensitive to gluten and you've been dismissed or disregarded by your doctor, you aren't alone. Standard laboratory testing often misses this all too common diagnosis, and it takes an average of ten years to get an accurate one.

Every person fits into one of four categories:

1. You have celiac disease and gluten causes an immune overreaction. You get bloated and gassy. Or maybe you get constipated, develop a rash, or feel anxious, depressed, or just plain tired. Approximately 1 percent of the U.S. population has celiac disease, but many are undiagnosed and many experts believe prevalence is higher.

2. You have nonceliac gluten sensitivity, which is more of an intolerance but shares several properties with celiac disease. Some research says up to 7 percent of the population suffers from it. You eat gluten and feel a reaction in your gut that may range from gurgling to diarrhea or swelling in the intestines. There are symptoms outside the gut too: perhaps you feel asocial and ineffective.[17]

3. You don't have either celiac disease or nonceliac gluten sensitivity, but you are one of the growing number of people who
   benefit from a gluten-free diet,[18] probably because you lack the
   enzymes needed to process wheat properly, as many people do.
   Your symptoms are mild, but when you eat gluten, you have
   bloating and weight gain, gas, or other signs of indigestion.

4. You have no reaction to gluten and do fine eating it (as far as
   you know; sometimes the reaction can be silent). I haven't
   met many of these people in the United States, but I met a
   few in France, where the wheat is more like what my great-
   grandmother ate.

Which one is your response to gluten? Based on my clinical experience, I imagine you fit into one of the first three categories and
need to go gluten free to see what's true for you.

Gluten problems used to be thought of as an allergy, but now we
know that there's an evolving and broad array of negative immune
reactions to the toxic family of gluten proteins found in wheat, rye,
barley, and their derivatives.

Because so many people fit along the broad spectrum of adverse
reactions to gluten, the World Health Organization has recommended screening the general population. I interpret their advice
to mean that you should remove all gluten and notice the benefits,
and then challenge yourself by adding gluten back into your food
plan, in a process called elimination/provocation. If you're struggling with weight and bloating, the chances are you'll get lean and
feel more energetic during the elimination phase.

### WHEAT BELLY: A BALANCED LOOK

**Lose the wheat, lose the weight.**

–WILLIAM DAVIS, M.D., WHEAT BELLY

*"Wheat belly," a term popularized by Dr. William Davis in his book
by the same title, describes the increase in visceral fat that gets*

*plunked down in your midsection and how it's linked to gluten
consumption.*

*My opinion is that this theory has some validity. While we don't
yet have solid evidence showing that everyone loses weight when
they remove gluten, I believe that many people develop leaky gut,
food intolerances, and fat-loss resistance from eating gluten. Gluten
is like a "gateway drug" to obesity. Many of my patients struggling
with weight try hard to eat healthy food, such as wheat bread. But
they don't realize that the gluten they are eating is actually punching
holes in their gut. Further, many women, particularly after age forty,
suffer from an intolerance to all grains, and gluten is particularly bad
news when it comes to getting lean.*

*Yet Dr. William Davis's book, which proposes eliminating wheat/
gluten from your diet, is not without controversy. Some people
point to the fact that the fiber found in wheat is an essential source
of nutrients and promotes growth of beneficial bacteria.[19] Others
say that people who eliminate wheat and gluten lose weight simply
because they are eating less.[20] The jury is still out. I like to go by your
symptoms. If you stop eating gluten for seventy-two hours and you
feel better, this is wonderful information to have.*

---

### From Dr. Sara's Case Files: Glenda, Age Seventy-One

- *Lost 19 pounds on the Hormone Reset Diet.*
- *Glenda has type 2 diabetes. Fasting blood sugars were 159 on the
  start day. After program completion: 82 mg/dL!*
- *Her hardest challenge was giving up grains. She craved sandwiches.*
- *"I went into this program reluctant and kind of doubting if I'd see
  any results. I have done a lot of diets in my lifetime, and this is
  the first program where I've ever lost significant belly fat. I never
  thought I would see my blood sugar down to two digits. I know
  that my doctor is going to be shocked and impressed. I would like*

*to maintain my results and lose even more belly fat. I'm so grateful for what I've achieved thus far."*

> **JUST SAY NO TO CEREAL**
>
> *It seems so harmless. Mornings are hectic, and it's simple to break out a box of cereal, feed it to the kids, and run out the door. But what is the cost of this convenience? Although it's an integral part of American culture, cereal isn't the friend that it might seem; in fact, cereal has been linked to nutrient deficiencies, broken digestion, and auto-immune diseases, and don't forget they contain opioids, which make them addictive.[21] Cereal doesn't have the protein you need and is often packed with sugar. It makes you more acidic and stressed. I'm not alone in my assessment of this favorite morning meal: a recent study proposed that cereal could be an environmental factor contributing to "diseases of affluence," like diabetes and obesity, because the human leptin system is not adapted to a cereal-based diet.[22]*
>
> *For breakfast, go for something that will help you feel energized throughout the day. Scrambled eggs with spinach, a smoothie with protein powder and greens, or non-GM tofu scrambled with veggies. If you must have sometime akin to cereal, try the recipe for porridge found on page 269.*

## The Vicious Cycle of Grains, Gluten, and Thyroid

When it comes to grains, they may increase your risk of thyroid problems such as autoimmunity, according to Dr. Datis Kharrazian, chiropractor and author of *Why Do I Still Have Thyroid Symptoms?* While it's well established that gluten sensitivity and celiac disease are more common in people with Hashimoto's disease, Dr.

Kharrazian ups the ante by suggesting that folks with slow thyroid function should go gluten free. The problem may be a case of mistaken identity: the protein in gluten resembles that of thyroid tissue. When gluten crosses the gut barrier, the immune system prepares for attack, and thyroid tissue gets caught in the battle. In one careful study of four hundred patients with autoimmune thyroiditis, 6 percent of them had antibodies in their blood to gliadin, the protein found in gluten.[23]

What's the safest bet? Stay off the grains and give your thyroid a break.

## Grain Free: The Three-Day Reset for Thyroid

If you've had symptoms for a while, or even if your grain intolerance has long gone undiagnosed, this reset could be just what you need to jump-start a whole new way of eating that supports, instead of breaks down, your belly's health. You might feel so good that you stay off grains after the twenty-one days of the Hormone Reset, depending on how much damage grains have inflicted upon you.

Dietary stress from certain foods, such as grains, is a major cause of weight-loss resistance, wreaking internal havoc on your best efforts at long-term fat loss. Removing grains for seventy-two hours helps shed the pounds and provide dramatic improvements in gut, pancreas, brain, and thyroid function, and it resets your insulin levels. This powerful three-day reset could be exactly what you need to give your organs a clean bill of health.

### GRAIN FREE RULES: DO THESE EACH DAY

Stock your pantry with enough foods that don't contain grain to sustain you for at least three days. Fortunately, it's much easier than it used to be ten or twenty years ago to find the grain-free foods that you need.

Here's what to do when going grain free, and remember to continue the rules you've already implemented from the previous resets:

1. **Avoid *all* grains, including flour** (even gluten-free). Stay away from the three Ps that cause Americans the most inflammation: pizza, pasta, and pastries. What specifically to avoid:

   • Bread, cereal, or other food made with any grains (even gluten-free).

   • Wheat, rye, barley, oat, corn, durum, millet, rice, spelt, or any type of grain flours or ingredients and byproducts made from those grains.

   • Processed foods containing grains, wheat, gluten derivatives, or thickeners. These foods include hot dogs, luncheon meats, mustard, pickles, ice cream, salad dressings, canned soups, dried soup mixes, nondairy creamers, processed cheeses, cream sauces, beer, spices, and hundreds of other common foods. Study labels to avoid chemicals.

   • Gluten-free carbohydrates. Don't trade gluten-filled refined carbohydrates for gluten-free refined carbohydrates. Studies show that refined carbohydrates, whether they contain gluten or not, increase your production of insulin, which blocks your ability to burn fat. Limit your carbohydrates so you can reduce insulin levels and permit greater fat burning.

   • Artificial seasonings and flavors. The food industry keeps these ingredients supersecret, so it's hard to know sometimes exactly what contains gluten. You *should* be suspicious. Look for ingredients like "seasoning," "flavoring," "natural flavoring," "hydrolyzed vegetable protein," "maltodextrin," and "modified food starch," which could be derived from wheat and contain gluten.

2. **Eat one pound of high-fiber vegetables per day.** For women, I recommend three to four cups of leafy greens such as kale,

broccoli, and lettuce. Approximately half should be lightly cooked and half should be raw, as in salads. This will be your main source of slow carbohydrates. They are slow carbs because they don't raise your insulin level and, as a result, don't make you store fat.

3. **Limit your net carbs**—that's total carbohydrates in grams minus fiber in grams—because those are the carbohydrates that raise your insulin levels and make you more likely to store fat. Women who need to lose weight should aim for 20 to 49 net carbs per day (see Net Carbohydrate Thresholds, page 81). The ideal limit on net carbs depends on your genetics and current metabolism; you will be able to add more net carbs after Day 21 (see chapter 11, where I recommend 50 to 99 net carbs per day for maintenance of your weight). You'll know the best carb threshold for you when you are losing weight (or maintaining your healthy weight) or losing fat and you don't suffer from carb cravings, plus your energy level is high. Listen to your body. The amount of carbs you can eat is highly variable.

4. **Eat clean proteins,** such as seafood, organic poultry, and eggs—approximately 8 to 12 ounces per day (about 80–110 grams). If they don't make you bloated and miserable, eat one half-cup per day of fresh or cooked beans.

5. **Eat only limited fresh fruits:** avocado, olives, and coconut. Avoid fruit juices and dried fruits.

### SWAPS FOR GRAINS

- Coconut wraps—these yummy alternatives to carb-filled tortillas are made from coconut meat and water.
- Romaine lettuce instead of bread or buns
- Coconut flour
- Baked sweet potatoes
- Kelp noodles
- If you're looking for a salty, crunchy experience, try roasted seaweed. It's a rich source of iodine and readily available at local

supermarkets and health food stores. I eat it when the rest of my
family is diving into the potato chips or wheat-based crackers.

• Flaxseed and dehydrated vegetable crackers

### SAMPLE MENU

Here is a suggested menu for resetting your thyroid, insulin, and
leptin by going grain free. For nutritional data, check out the Notes
section.[24]

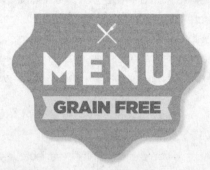

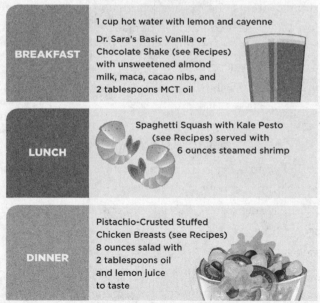

**BREAKFAST**
1 cup hot water with lemon and cayenne

Dr. Sara's Basic Vanilla or Chocolate Shake (see Recipes) with unsweetened almond milk, maca, cacao nibs, and 2 tablespoons MCT oil

**LUNCH**
Spaghetti Squash with Kale Pesto (see Recipes) served with 6 ounces steamed shrimp

**DINNER**
Pistachio-Crusted Stuffed Chicken Breasts (see Recipes) 8 ounces salad with 2 tablespoons oil and lemon juice to taste

## Supplements

Now that you're determined to go grain free and unlock your metabolism, vitamin D may kill two birds with one stone. The first bird: it boosts thyroid function, creating a welcoming environment for you to lose weight. The second bird: it is linked to better blood glucose regulation.[25] This helps with blood sugar spikes and keeps the lid on overeating. I recommend a dose of 2,000 to 4,000 IU per day.

## Cell to Soul Practice

Eliminating grains can be difficult in a world brimming with bread, cookies, and other yummy baked goods. It's easy to be drawn to these foods when you are feeling low, tired, or even happy. (I mean, who hasn't rewarded herself with a cookie?) However, I'm convinced that when you see how good you feel by eliminating grains, you will be motivated to stick with it. It also fires up your intention and behaviors to do a ritual of release. This can be a powerful and subtle way to affirm your commitment, release your desire for refined carbs, and start your reset on the right foot.

Look at going grain free as an opportunity to let go of things in your life that aren't serving you. Is that morning muffin making you feel energized and joyful throughout the day? I think not. I like to do a spiritual ritual of letting go that is particularly suited to this reset. Use this one, or choose other objects and places that might speak to you:

Go to a body of water with a piece of bread. Stand at the edge of the water for a few minutes, reflecting on what you want to release into the water. Slowly break pieces off the bread (warning: overt symbolism alert!) and imagine yourself, with each piece, letting go of things that don't serve you anymore. Watch the bread float away. Observe how you feel. Lighter? Relieved? Joyful?

There is no single way to let go. You might try this variation of the fisherman's prayer as you learn to let go and yield to the universe: "Dear Lord, be good to me. The sea is so wide, and my boat is so small."

## Exercise

We need to bust some serious belly fat in this seventy-two-hour reset. Your main enemy with fat loss is the metabolically active brew known collectively as your visceral fat, located in your abdomen. It works against your goal to lose weight and fit into your skinny jeans because it is the epicenter of the inflammation we've been discussing.

If your solution is hitting the treadmill 24/7, think again. The varying views on this topic might surprise you. Some believe that aerobic exercise might not be effective at reducing this fat,[26] while other folks believe exercise is essential.[27] Personally, I'm not that impressed with the power of exercise to get me into my jeans. Most research shows that exercise is only about 4 to 20 percent of the story when it comes to fat loss. We also know that less is more. That's why I got inspired by Gretchen Reynolds's scientific 7-Minute Workout,[28] and I decided to modify it for myself and other women who shouldn't be doing squats (one word: hemorrhoids!). It's short and sweet yet provides you with a great way to get a high-intensity workout. Research shows that it can have similar, if not better, effects than a longer workout. What's not to love?

The 7-Minute scientific workout is now available in the original and an advanced version, both online and in a free app.[29] Just skip the squat and replace it with another plank or wall sit.

## Test Yourself

Are you wondering if you need to reassess your relationship with grains? There are a few ways to test yourself: by eliminating grains in this reset and seeing what happens when you add them back into your diet (for reintroducing grains, see chapter 10), by testing your blood for an immune reaction, or by testing your genes (usually with a saliva test).

If you're interested in testing your blood, talk to your doctor about measuring your antibodies against the proteins found in gluten. The two best tests that I recommend are the Cyrex and the ALCAT.

### YOGA BREATHING FOR YOUR THYROID

*Boost your body and spirit with a simple exercise that yogis have done for millennia, the chin lock, also known in Sanskrit transliteration as* **Jalandhara Bandha***. This is thought to stimulate the thyroid, while the breathing also calms and centers your mind.*

*Start in a comfortable cross-legged position, breathing in and out through your nose. On an inhalation, hold your breath and lower your chin so that it's "locked" in (or toward) that little indented space in your neck. Hold for ten seconds and then, while you're still holding your breath, raise your head. Slowly exhale through your nose. Breathe normally for a few breaths. Repeat the sequence four more times, resting in between each repetition.*

## Notes from Hormone Resetters

"I lost 18 pounds. I feel better than I have in months and have been sleeping better than I have in years. I had no idea that food could be my culprit in making me feel so bad." —*Donna*

"I really liked the very subtle approach to removing foods from your daily habits. I found that as I got used to not having a certain food, it was time to remove another, never really feeling like I was going without. I was about 60 pounds overweight, and I lost 20 during this detox. I am planning on continuing for a little while longer, just to solidify my new food code, which is to eat fresh, raw, and nonprocessed, [and] also to limit alcohol, caffeine, and red meat. I couldn't be happier with this process and my results." —*Craig*

"My husband and I couldn't figure out why the Paleo diet that worked so well for him was not a good fit for me. I gained weight, and my hormones got all out of whack, while he turned into Captain America. One day he heard an interview with Dr. Sara Gottfried on one of his favorite podcasts and shared with me the impressive work she had been doing helping women cure their hormone woes. Her [Hormone Reset] was the answer. It took me exactly where I needed to go and has empowered me to stay on track and keep improving my health long after the end of the program. I lost 2 inches of scary abdominal fat from my waist, restored my sleep, reduced anxiety, and gained a ton of resources, confidence, and some beautiful daily rituals." —*Melanie*

## Final Word

Good luck with the Grain Free reset. No one can tell you how it will make you feel. Give yourself the gift of curiosity and sacred self-experimentation. With all the talking heads discussing the pros and cons of grains, find out what is true for you, your body, and the bathroom scale. After three days, take a few moments of quiet time to reflect on how you feel emotionally and physically. Put your hand on your belly, feel the warmth of your hand sending a healing vibe to your long-suffering gut, and take in the love and healing. It's a powerful retooling for your body, and I often see amazing results in just three days.

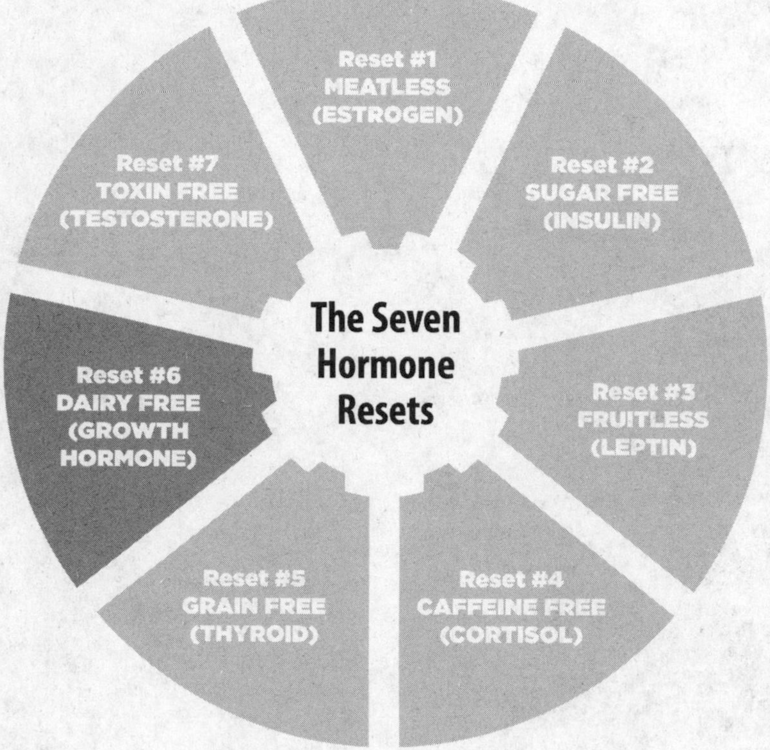

The Seven Hormone Resets

Reset #1
MEATLESS
(ESTROGEN)

Reset #2
SUGAR FREE
(INSULIN)

Reset #3
FRUITLESS
(LEPTIN)

Reset #4
CAFFEINE FREE
(CORTISOL)

Reset #5
GRAIN FREE
(THYROID)

Reset #6
DAIRY FREE
(GROWTH
HORMONE)

Reset #7
TOXIN FREE
(TESTOSTERONE)

# CHAPTER 8

# Dairy Free

GROWTH HORMONE RESET: *Days 16 to 18*

There is a good reason you aren't getting thin, despite your skinny lattes, nonfat cottage cheese, and nonfat fro-yos. These items that you *think* will lead to weight loss might actually be promoting weight gain. Despite your best intentions, your daily dairy could be making you fat.

That's because dairy is one of the top foods that contribute to excess inflammation, a state that causes you to gain weight and become resistant to losing it. Remember that inflammation is your body's emergency response system, a normal part of what your body does. When your body is functioning properly, inflammation should stop after seventy-two hours. But when prolonged, it's a problem that I call "biochemistry gone wrong." The impact of inflammation cannot be overstated. It's a major contributor to obesity, among many other diseases.

By eliminating this irritant to the immune system, you will be amazed at how quickly you'll get results. In addition to seeing a reduction in symptoms like fatigue, irritable bowel, anxiety, and even tight jeans, you'll lose weight as your body's inflammation subsides and your misfiring hormones go back into balance. I was stunned to learn that when I added one serving of dairy, after cutting it out for two weeks, I gained 3 pounds overnight—probably because my gut became inflamed and bloated, and I retained fluid.

With the Dairy Free three-day reset, you may be able to determine if dairy is what's holding you back from reaching your ideal weight.

## Self-Assessment

Do you have or have you experienced in the past six months . . .

☐ A swelling of the lips, tongue, face, throat, or mouth?

☐ A gurgling belly after a hunk of cheese or bowl of ice cream?

☐ Bloating or an irritable bowel?

☐ The feeling that a meal without cheese is a meal not worth having?

☐ Diarrhea or constipation after make-your-own-sundae night?

☐ An addiction to a milk-based treat, such as a latte or Frappuccino?

☐ A stuffy or runny nose, watery or itchy eyes, coughing, sneezing, or wheezing after ingesting an afternoon yogurt?

☐ Frequent skin reactions, such as a rash, itchy bumps or hives, or red skin?

☐ An unsettling feeling like you are addicted to your favorite cheeses? A habit of being glued to the cheese station at parties?

☐ A tendency toward sinusitis (sinus infection), but you have never figured out why?

☐ A memory of having a rash in reaction to cow's milk as a baby, but your mom told you that you outgrew it as you got older?

☐ Anaphylaxis—a sudden and severe allergic reaction during which you can have trouble breathing, talking, or swallowing due to swelling?

*Interpret Your Results*

- **If you have five or more of these symptoms,** you are very likely intolerant of or allergic to dairy. The inflammation caused by dairy might be your roadblock to the size you want to be. Please read this chapter so you can reduce or eliminate your symptoms and lose weight. You may also want to consider getting yourself tested, as described later in this chapter (page 191).

- **If you have fewer than five of these symptoms or are unsure,** I recommend following this reset and seeing how your body reacts to three days without dairy.

---

### From Dr. Sara's Case Files: Gina, Age Fifty

---

- *Lost 14 pounds.*
- *Hardest to give up were bread and cheese.*
- *"I have been overweight my entire life and know I am a STRESS EATER. I was able to lose 14 pounds, and I realized for the first time how empowered I felt. I never felt hungry, which made the process easy for me. I didn't put a lot of thought into the 'I can't do this'; rather I took it day by day and watched the pounds drop off. It gave me the tools to look at my diet in a whole new way. My 14-year-old son said to me: 'Mom, I am going to choose to eat healthy. You have been an inspiration to me.' That was the best gift of all."*

---

## The Science Behind Dairy Free

Humans' love affair with dairy starts at birth. A mother's breast milk is clearly known as the healthiest form of food for her child.

We're designed for human breast milk, but cow's milk? The jury is still out. In fact, humans are the only mammals that drink milk as adults. Time to rethink it? Most people—approximately 75 percent, including most people of African, Native American, and Asian descent—can't make lactase, the enzyme that breaks down dairy, as they get older and therefore can't tolerate dairy. Northern Europeans fare somewhat better and are more likely to keep making lactase as they age.

The bottom line is that dairy (along with gluten) is one of most common hidden food sensitivities. Dairy sensitivity is the result of long-term yet subtle violence against your gut. Maybe you took antibiotics for acne as a kid, or perhaps you take ibuprofen for a nagging injury. Quite feasibly, stress has been your constant companion. Or maybe you like to golf and have been exposed to endocrine-disrupting pesticides on the golf course. These small insults add up to create leaky gut. This syndrome makes food particles, such as the proteins in dairy, trigger an alarm in the immune system of your gut. Now you have a food sensitivity and low-grade but pathological inflammation—and it can make you fat, insulin resistant, congested, tired, foggy, depressed, asthmatic, and cranky.

If you think you are the only one cursed with a future devoid of ice cream sundaes and cheese plates, think again. Dairy allergies, reduced enzymes to break down lactose (the main sugar in milk), and sensitivities are on the rise.[1] As you can see in the figure on the opposite page, half of adults who are sensitive to gluten are also sensitive to dairy!

## Dairy Causes Inflammation in Susceptible People

Inflammation is your body's natural defense system: when bad guys invade, your white blood cells kick into gear and send chemicals called cytokines to protect you. But when inflammation shifts into overdrive and gets imbalanced, it can become the cause of many other diseases, including cancer, diabetes, dementia, and (as I've

# The Dairy Stats

| | |
|---|---|
| Adults with dairy intolerance worldwide | 75% |
| U.S. adults with dairy intolerance | 25–33% |
| African Americans with reduced enzymes to digest milk (lactose intolerance) | 75–80% |
| Asian Americans with lactose intolerance | 90% |
| Native Americans with lactose intolerance | 100% |
| Mexican Americans with lactose intolerance | 53% |
| Adults who are sensitive to gluten who also are sensitive to dairy | 50% |

already mentioned) obesity. Any inflammation lasting longer than seventy-two hours is a problem and will start to poison you and your health.

Unfortunately, women are more vulnerable to inflammation than men, so we need to be even more careful—that is, women of all ages have more robust immune responses to invaders (bugs, vaccines, and food) than men, which leads to higher rates in women of autoimmunity, thyroid issues, infections, arthritis, oral health problems, and other conditions.[2] The reasons are not fully understood but may be linked to our lower levels of testosterone and higher levels of estrogen.[3]

As Ann Wigmore, author, holistic health advocate, and nutrition-ist, says, "The food you eat can be either the safest and most power-ful form of medicine or the slowest form of poison." Inflammation is poison when it doesn't resolve, like a smoldering fire in your gut that makes you leaky, bloated, and gassy, and it causes trouble when you want to lose weight. Fortunately, it doesn't always require a lengthy doctor visit to reclaim your health and weight; it just takes kicking inflammation to the curb by changing what you put on your fork. With my Dairy Free reset, you are giving yourself the chance to put out that fire and start anew.

### YOUR ACIDIC SUPERHIGHWAY: WISE ADVICE FROM KRIS CARR

One of the key reasons we're inflamed, feel off, and can't lose weight is that we drive every day on the acid superhighway. What's the major contributor to your high acid level? **Dairy.** Fasten your seatbelts, because I've got good news: you can fix that problem very easily by creating a proper pH, which reflects acid-alkaline balance in your own body.

Here's the rundown: The pH scale runs from 0 to 14. Neutral pH is 7. A pH greater than 7 is alkaline, while a pH lower than 7 is acidic. "An understanding of how to keep your blood in an alkaline range is important for maintaining good health," says Kris Carr, **New York Times** bestselling author of **Crazy Sexy Kitchen.** Kris works with a large community of raving fans to balance their pH levels for opti-mum health and harmony. (You can find her at http://kriscarr.com.)

Your body doesn't just magically find pH balance; it works ex-tremely hard to create it so that your biochemistry works optimally. When you make poor lifestyle choices or are burdened by toxins, your body has to work even harder. For good health, your body needs to be slightly alkaline. Carr explains that the Standard American Diet, which includes coffee, dairy, sugar, fried foods, soda, artificial sweeteners,

and simple carbs, sabotages your chance at pH balance. "Most folks
are bathing their cells in an acid bath by making poor choices three or
more times per day," explains Kris. "A menu like this keeps the body in
panic mode all day, every day." This takes a toll on the body, especially
on the digestive system, liver, and kidneys. "Inflammation, allergies,
arthritis, skin problems, mood disorders, depression, constipation,
bowel issues, stress (physical and mental), and chronic disease love
this diet," she says.

Kris's recommendation? Banish an acidic diet that is high in animal
products (dairy included), processed carbs, refined sugar, booze, cigarettes, and coffee. Replace this with a more alkaline diet, consisting of
leafy greens, wheatgrass, veggies, sprouts, avocados, green smoothies, and soups to flood your body with chlorophyll, enzymes, vitamins,
minerals, and oxygen. "Look at your plate. Peek in your glass," says
Carr. "What direction are you moving in? Burger, fries, diet cola, muffin, candy bar? Acid bath! Green drinks, salads, sprouts, wheatgrass?
Alkaline super disco! Your goal is to make energy deposits instead of
constant withdrawals."[4]

Enough said. Be like Kris and dump the dairy. Your pH will thank you.

----

# The Case Against Casein

If you feel burpy, belchy, or bloated after you eat dairy, you may have
a sensitivity to casein, a protein in milk. Casein is a leading cause
of inflammation among my clients who are overweight or obese.
With this protein, we have yet another case of mistaken identity.
Remember the problem of gluten and how it punches holes in your
gut (the leaky gut) and how your immune system fights back with
its weapon of choice, the antibody? It's the same sad story here with
dairy. Your sensitivity to dairy occurs when your immune system
falsely identifies the dairy protein as harmful and inappropriately
fires off allergic antibodies for protection. This interaction triggers

a cascade of body chemicals that set off the fire throughout your body and make you hang on to weight. These chemicals include histamine, which causes symptoms that may include

- a swelling of the lips, mouth, tongue, face, or throat;
- skin reactions, such as hives, a rash, or red, itchy skin; or
- a stuffy or runny nose, sinusitis, sneezing, itchy eyes, coughing, or wheezing.

The most serious reaction to a milk allergy can involve anaphylaxis, a potentially life-threatening reaction that can occur rapidly. Food allergies (including casein in milk) are believed to be the leading cause of anaphylaxis outside the hospital setting. People who have asthma in addition to a serious food allergy to a protein, such as casein, are at greater risk for worse outcomes if they suffer an exposure and develop an anaphylactic reaction. Symptoms such as swelling inside your mouth, chest pain, hives, or difficulty breathing within minutes of consuming a milk product may mean you are experiencing an anaphylactic reaction and need emergency medical attention. Most of us won't experience this scary phenomenon. But some of us will just feel bad, fat, and bloated after eating dairy.

## Be Wary of Whey

Remember Little Miss Muffet, eating her curds and whey? Ever wonder what the heck that whey stuff was? Whey is the "serum" of milk—the liquid remaining after milk has been curdled and strained. It's used to make processed foods, such as bread, crackers, and pastry, as well as cheeses, such as ricotta. In modern times, Little Miss Muffet has to be careful not to eat too much whey, or she might get renamed Little Miss Muffin Top. While whey intolerance may not be as severe as casein, it's still common.

If milk gives you the sniffles and a gurgling tummy, it might not be due to the casein. You may have a whey allergy or sensitivity, another type of immune overreaction caused by dairy. In the Western diet, dairy protein consists of mostly casein and approximately 20 percent whey. Some folks experience double trouble and are allergic to both casein and whey. Overall, whey protein leads to fewer allergies than casein. But for those who have a reaction to milk, whey may be the secret culprit because it is often dried into a powder and added to foods and supplements that you wouldn't expect to contain dairy.

Can you be allergic to casein but not whey, or vice versa? Yes. The symptoms of both allergies are similar. I find that some of my patients, especially those who've been drinking smoothies made with whey protein powder for a while, develop a whey allergy. How do you know? The two Rs: *remove* and then *reintroduce*. For one week, stop eating anything with whey in the ingredients. See how you feel. For the second week, stop eating all dairy. See how you feel and compare that feeling with the first week. This is a great way to cultivate your body awareness!

## A Line on Lactose Intolerance

Another potential reason you may have symptoms when you consume dairy is lactose intolerance. You may have friends who drink Lactaid milk or take enzymes before eating a dairy product. That's because they are lactose intolerant, which means they lack sufficient enzymes to digest the main sugar in milk, called lactose.

A lactose intolerance is usually milder than a casein or whey intolerance, which as we've learned can cause hives and difficulty breathing in its most severe form. Still, it's a major nuisance: when you can't fully digest the lactose in dairy products, you get a civil war in your small intestine. The battlefield in your belly often appears later in life, with symptoms including gurgling, bloating, discomfort, gas, diarrhea, or gastroesophageal reflux (GERD). How do you know if you've got it? Ask your health professional for one of the following tests:[5]

*Hydrogen breath test.* The preferred way to test for lactose intolerance, this test is based on the measurement of how much hydrogen you exhale after breathing into a balloon-like container.

*Lactose tolerance test.* This test examines your gut's reaction to a liquid that contains high levels of lactose. Two hours after drinking the liquid with lactose, a blood test measures the amount of glucose in your bloodstream. If your glucose level doesn't rise, it means your body isn't properly digesting the lactose-rich drink.

*Stool acidity test.* When babies or children can't do the two previous tests, the acidity in the stool can be measured as fecal pH. When you consume dairy, fermentation of undigested lactose produces acids that can be detected in a stool sample. As described earlier in this chapter, dairy is acid forming, and when you cannot digest lactose, you create even more acidity (measured as low pH).

By now, you won't be surprised to learn that there is a genetic tendency to have lactose intolerance. Unfortunately, a dairy intolerance—whether it's casein, whey, or lactose—may mean that you are at risk for other health problems too. Drinking your beloved milk may increase your chance of diabetes, although debate continues.[6] And research shows that a cow's milk allergy increases your risk of mental health problems, like schizophrenia.[7] So, if you do suffer from a milk allergy, be aware of these correlations and pay attention to changes in your health.

THE MILK MYTH

Most of us were raised to think that milk is required for strong bones. In 2005, the U.S. Department of Agriculture told us to drink three servings of low-fat milk each day—mostly because milk provides calcium, potassium, and vitamin D (which is added to milk). The rationale is that milk will help reduce bone fractures and blood pressure.

We've all seen the commercials: it does a body good, right? Maybe not. A growing number of experts believe that milk is a top allergen, the cause of many symptoms, such as constipation, sinusitis, rashes, bloating, and irritable bowel syndrome.

Given the number of people I see in my practice who are intolerant to dairy, I agree with a professor at Harvard School of Public Health, Walter Willett, M.D., Ph.D., who calls the milk recommendation a "step in the wrong direction." It turns out that there's very little science to prove milk consumption reduces your risk of bone fractures. Luckily, you don't need to drink milk to have strong bones. Alternative sources of calcium include salmon, sardines, turnip greens, almonds, kale, bok choy, broccoli, spinach, and sweet potatoes.

If you are indeed intolerant to casein, whey, or lactose, don't worry. Despite the convincing commercials from the industry, a panel of experts found that dairy is not essential to a healthy diet.[8]

----

# The Addictive Side of Dairy

Did a friend ever have to literally pull you away from the frozen yogurt shop? When the cheese plate comes at dinner, do you elbow others out of the way and make a beeline for it? There is a reason you feel "addicted" to your favorite dairy treats. It turns out that they contain "casomorphins," protein fragments that come from the digestion of the milk protein casein. A cousin of morphine and heroin, casomorphins are opioids that keep you addicted. Casomorphins are like crack, which is why so many of us have an addiction to cheese or lattes or cream in our coffee. With its drug-like effects, no wonder dairy is constipating, just like opiate painkillers. Overall, dairy is low in fiber and slows down digestion.

It's good to have this information so you can understand your emotional and physical relationship to dairy foods. It can be tempting to turn to your addictive foods when you're feeling under pressure, down, or just plain bored. While food can be soothing, it's important to remember that it's not a salve for stress. Interestingly, more than 90 percent of your body's genetic expression—in other words, how those lovely genes play out or manifest for you—is determined by what you eat. You consume more than one ton of food per year, so this is a ton (literally and figuratively) of information for your genes.

How do you want to influence your genes? Feed them morphine-like substances or kale?[9] By choosing to eliminate dairy from your diet, even for seventy-two hours, you could be doing your body a wonderful service to clear your addictions and begin with a clean slate.

## The Link Between Dairy and Growth Hormone

You didn't think I'd stop talking about hormones, did you? Let's get to the effect of dairy on your hormones. It turns out that conventional dairy raises growth hormone and insulin. And growth hormone, along with cortisol, determines how much fat you deposit on your belly.[10] Like cortisol, insulin, and all the other hormones of metabolism, growth hormone should be in the neutral zone for optimal functioning: not too high and not too low.

The problem is that synthetic growth hormone, known as "bovine somatotropin," has been on the market since 1994 and is injected into about a third of the nation's nine million dairy cows.[11] When injected once every two weeks, the hormone can increase a cow's milk output by 10 to 15 percent.[12] You don't need to be a scientist to figure out that if cows are injected with growth hormone to fatten them and you eat their products, you may also be affected.

Avoid dairy beginning with this three-day reset and for the remainder of your Hormone Reset, and if you pass the reentry test (chapter 10), buy organic dairy from cows without growth hormone.

The illustration below presents a balanced look at the pros, cons, and unsettled science of dairy. For citations, go to www.Hormone Reset.com/bonus.

# DAIRY: The Scorecard

## PRO

- May lower your chance of kidney stones.
- Tastes creamy and good.

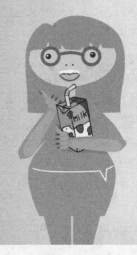

## CON

- During World War II, when dairy and meat were rationed, heart disease rates fell and Americans were healthier than now.
- Paradoxically, may increase your risk of fractures. It's not proven that dairy itself is necessary for bone health.
- Most conventional dairy contains growth hormones and is ultra-pasteurized, which kills off the good bacteria.
- Contributes to rising rates of allergies, intolerances, and sensitivities—particularly to casein, whey, and lactose.
- May increase your risk of breast cancer, but data are mixed.
- Linked to increased mortality in men and women.
- No benefit to body weight or fat loss.

## Dairy Free: The Three-Day Reset for Growth Hormone

You've now had a chance to see how good you feel after the three-day eliminations of conventional meat, sugar, fruit, caffeine, and grain. Now it's time to heal further from going dairy free. In only three days you can reduce inflammation, reset your growth hormone and insulin balanced, and determine if dairy is making it impossible to lose weight.

Remember that you want to keep your eyes on the prize—getting lean for the long term. You now have the finish line in sight! Only six more days to go before you begin to add back one challenge food at a time, to track your biological response to it.

In the Dairy Free reset, you'll be able to swap out your favorites with creamy but nondairy choices. My hunch is that with some creativity, you won't even miss your milky companions.

### DAIRY FREE RULES: DO THESE EACH DAY

When you eliminate dairy, you'll make more room for alkaline-forming foods filled with fiber, minerals, and iron. Remember to continue the rules you've already implemented from the previous resets.

1. **Avoid milk, cheese, butter, kefir, and yogurt.**
2. **Make sure you are getting enough protein** in the form of crustaceans, cold-water fish, grass-fed beef, pastured eggs, seeds, and maybe beans (if they don't cause weight gain).
3. **Eat lots of fiber and fresh vegetables** to fill you up. Continue to aim for one pound of vegetables per day, or even more.
4. **Drink "milk"**—just not from an animal (see Milk Alternatives on page 187).
5. **Substitute conventional butter with pastured ghee,** which has the milk solids removed and is casein free.

6. **Make creamy non-dairy soups** that will last three days.

7. **Look for foods that are labeled "vegan"** at your supermarket or your local health food store; this means they contain no dairy. Examples include "vegannaise" and nondairy cheeses. Just be sure to check the labels to ensure they don't have casein. For instance, on page 279, you'll find a recipe for crusted chicken stuffed with almond cheese and roasted red pepper. Yum!

### SAMPLE MENU

A suggested dairy-free menu for resetting your insulin and growth hormone is on the following page. For nutritional data, check out the Notes section.[13]

### MILK ALTERNATIVES

*If you can't have your tall glass of cow's milk, you still have a plethora of other options.*

- *Almond milk. Great in smoothies or with your favorite (gluten-free) cookie. Make sure to buy unsweetened so you bypass the extra sugar.*
- *Coconut milk. Made from healthful coconuts, this milk has a distinct taste that can be great whether you drink it alone or use it for cooking. Scrumptious in shakes!*
- *Hemp milk. This is another milk in your arsenal when you are eliminating dairy from your diet. Hemp protein is one of the most digestible if you have gut issues.*
- *Coconut kefir. This product is gluten- and dairy-free—and it's a great source of fermented food. Go to www.cocokefir.com, or make your own version.[14]*

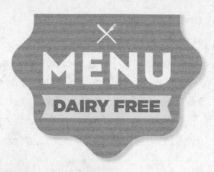

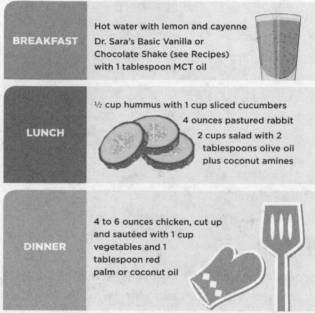

**BREAKFAST**
Hot water with lemon and cayenne
Dr. Sara's Basic Vanilla or Chocolate Shake (see Recipes) with 1 tablespoon MCT oil

**LUNCH**
½ cup hummus with 1 cup sliced cucumbers
4 ounces pastured rabbit
2 cups salad with 2 tablespoons olive oil plus coconut amines

**DINNER**
4 to 6 ounces chicken, cut up and sautéed with 1 cup vegetables and 1 tablespoon red palm or coconut oil

## Supplements

Digestive enzymes can help lessen inflammation, and I encourage you to take them. We all make fewer enzymes as we age, so popping a few digestive enzymes before a meal can really help after age forty. Lactase can be taken as a chewable pill that helps you digest lactose if you're intolerant,[15] but my preference always is to get to the root cause, which may be imbalanced gut bacteria. You can also take digestive enzymes that help you break down casein.

## Cell to Soul Practice

We all have to eat. But according to yoga's sister science, ayurveda, it's more important to pay attention to *how* you eat than *what* you eat. Personally, I believe both are important, but I respect this message from the sages of ayurveda, and you should too. Here's the idea: mindful eating promotes good digestion. In modern life, it's easy to scarf down a meal at your desk or in your car. I notice that sometimes I start to clear the plates from the dinner table at home before we are even finished! For this reset, focus on eating as a spiritual practice. Not only does this improve your digestion, it also gives you the opportunity to stay present to your experience.

Here are a few basic ayurvedic rules to follow:

- Don't drink water during a meal; this dissipates the "digestive fire" you need.
- Eat your biggest meals in the middle of the day, when your digestion is strongest.
- Eat according to your state. For instance, if you are feeling tired, eat foods with spices for a little boost. If you are feeling spacey, eat grounding foods like warm vegetable soup.
- Don't eat while reading or watching television, which distracts from the meditative nature of your meal.
- Rest after eating to allow your gut to assimilate nutrients.

## Exercise

The right kind of exercise can reset your metabolic hormones to healthy levels, and we know this is important for getting lean. Most people think that exercising for forty-five minutes, continuously and at a moderate pace, will help them shed pounds. The research shows otherwise. Women don't lose weight after sticking to this exercise regimen for three months![16]

When your metabolism is broken by leaky gut and inflammation, one of the fastest ways to fix it is with interval training—which to me is a prescription to exercise like a cavewoman. Sprinting intermittently, followed by moderate exercise, works superbly to reset growth hormone, insulin, and cortisol. Most people refer to this form of movement as high-intensity interval training (HIIT), which is proven to work for overweight women.[17] A recent meta-analysis of ten studies, which included 273 patients with heart conditions and a broken metabolism, showed that HIIT has double the benefit in terms of fitness compared with moderate-intensity continuous training.[18]

HIIT is a system of interval training that's superefficient, with multiple rounds of high-intensity burst training interspersed with less intense exercises.[19] The idea is to do it for a minimum of twenty-five to thirty minutes four days per week.

Here are a few pointers for how to do HIIT:

- Warm up for five minutes with your favorite type of exercise.

- Run for one minute, then briskly walk or jog for two minutes. If you can't jog or run, walk as fast as you can for one minute, then walk at a less intense but still brisk pace for two minutes. Repeat this sequence for twenty-five to thirty minutes. Or you can try biking: do a five-minute warm-up, then cycle hard, with your highest possible effort, interspersed with a more moderate effort every other minute. After fifteen minutes, pedal backward for three minutes and then repeat the sequence.

- Finish your workout with at least five minutes of active stretching.

According to the founders, HIIT naturally releases HGH (human growth hormone), which helps you burn fat and gain lean muscle.[20] From my personal experience, it works, but science is also in total agreement: HIIT is *way* better than running or stepping for an hour!

## Test Yourself

When it comes to looking at your reaction to dairy, there are several tests to consider.

- Take the hydrogen breath test (described earlier in the chapter, page 182), which will most accurately assess lactose intolerance.
- Measure your IGF-1 (insulin-like growth factor 1), which is an approximation of your growth hormone level.

There are limitations to these tests, and they are best interpreted in the context of the rest of your health with a knowledgeable practitioner.

## Notes from Hormone Resetters

"I think the most surprising thing for me was how much I've enjoyed the experience. I just didn't have cravings. Having that 'craving stress' removed made eating healthy things more of a pleasure and also made implementing other things like exercise, sleep, and daily habits easier. Even though I considered myself a healthy eater before, I have a different relationship with food now." —*Kirsten*

"I entered the program because I was fatigued, depressed, and obese. I kept remembering Dr. Gottfried's quote, paraphrasing someone else, that imperfect action trumps perfect inaction. So I began the journey. While I experience more peace, more energy, have lost 14 pounds with no difficulty and with no cravings, the greatest gift has been that of an increased feeling of well-being. I'd say to anyone who learns about this program that the time spent in preparation and the time spent detoxing will change your life significantly. And I believe that the gains made with this journey are ones that are sustainable. The materials are so incredible. Just reading them and absorbing them are like taking a postgraduate course in how to care for soul, mind, and body." —*Anna*

"I was stunned with my weight loss, and that really wasn't why I was interested in the journey. I lost 12 pounds and 3 inches off my waist and 3 inches off my hips. My sleep improved, which was my overall goal. And I have felt so much calmer and at peace with myself. I feel like I have found my premenopausal self again." —*Deborah*

## Final Word

Dairy can feel healing. Think of a glass of milk before bed, perhaps with a sprinkle of cinnamon. Some people are fine when they consume dairy from high-quality sources, but the important takeaway of this reset is that dairy cravings and addiction are real, allergies and intolerances are on the rise, and both aspects may be contributing to your weight gain.

Dairy contains biochemical and emotional triggers of craving and addiction. Milk features L-tryptophan, which converts in the body to serotonin, the feel-good brain chemical, and melatonin, the sleep hormone. Milk also has choline, which has a soothing effect. Nature designed milk to contain casomorphins to help young mammals engage in nursing and adapt, yet modern milk production has increased your exposure to the opiate-like qualities far in excess of what was intended for the human species. Cow milk contains about seven times as much casein as human breast milk. Cheese requires approximately ten pounds of milk to produce one pound of cheese. That's a lot of casein and casomorphin exposure. No wonder dairy can feel addictive.

If that's not enough to encourage you to dump dairy for three days and the rest of the Hormone Reset Diet, consider this: because cows tend to be milked most of the year, they are often pregnant. In the final stage of gestation, cow milk (even organic) contains 33 times as much estrogen as milk from nonpregnant cows. You know from the first reset that estrogen pollution is on the rise; now it's time to remove dairy in order to continue the aggregate hormone reset.

However, to get to the point of using dairy wisely, many of us need to take a step back before we take a step forward. This means a reset. Just like you reboot your computer every once in a while to make it work more efficiently, you can benefit from doing the same for your body. So, if you love your afternoon tea with a dash of milk or your morning Greek yogurt, this is not good-bye forever. It's more like "See you later." Commit to going dairy free, and then congratulate yourself. When you put your energy into this reset, you are giving yourself a chance for a new chapter in your book of dairy.

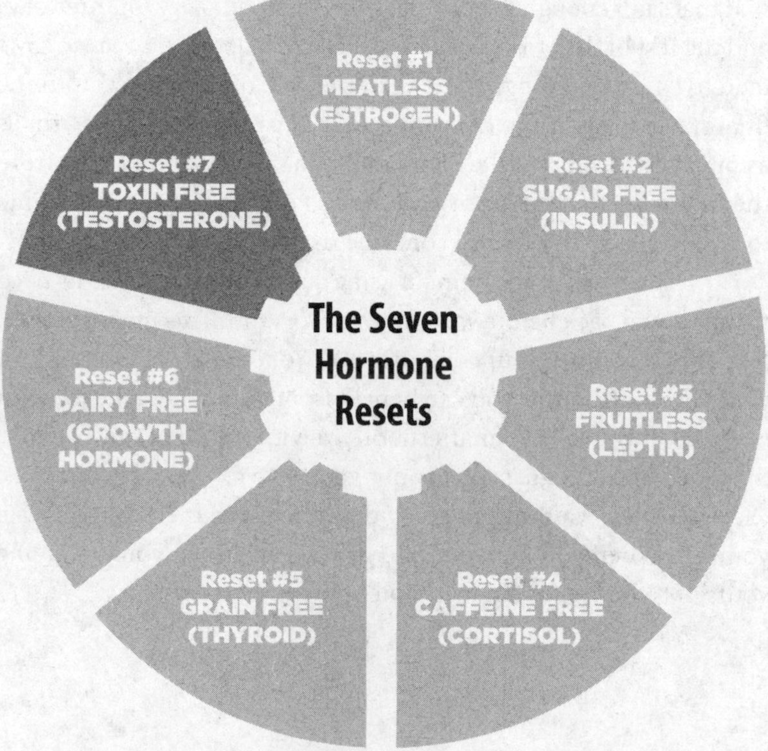

The Seven Hormone Resets

Reset #1
MEATLESS
(ESTROGEN)

Reset #2
SUGAR FREE
(INSULIN)

Reset #3
FRUITLESS
(LEPTIN)

Reset #4
CAFFEINE FREE
(CORTISOL)

Reset #5
GRAIN FREE
(THYROID)

Reset #6
DAIRY FREE
(GROWTH
HORMONE)

Reset #7
TOXIN FREE
(TESTOSTERONE)

# CHAPTER 9

# Toxin Free

Imagine a world in which you follow every rule for good health. You've cut out meat and alcohol, sugar, high-fructose fruit, caffeine, grain, and dairy. You diligently exercise for thirty minutes four days per week. You manage your stress through yoga and meditation, have a close network of friends, and express your feelings. No need for a detox, right?

*Wrong.* Even with our best efforts, we become toxic simply because of the world in which we live. Our blood is full of toxins; scientists call it "body burden."

The unsettling truth is that environmental exposure is on the rise. Most food you eat is probably genetically modified (GM) and sprayed with pesticides and fertilizers. Even if you're careful to avoid genetically modified food at home, when you go out to a restaurant, you might order steak from a cow raised on GM feed and injected with synthetic hormones. Not only is your food toxic, there are harmful chemicals in cosmetics as well. The average woman applies 515 synthetic chemicals in a *single day*.[1] Even the water you drink and your household cleaning products could be toxic. Our toxic surroundings not only usher in the risk of certain diseases, but also make you resistant to losing weight. If you're overweight, you're toxic by definition because endocrine disruptors are stored in your fat cells. In short, this is again biochemistry gone wrong.

But all hope is not lost. I believe that when we create the optimal conditions, the body will naturally heal. That's why detoxification is so powerful: it can flip the switch toward healing, repair, and fat loss. Along the way, you can uncover the innate intelligence of your body and soul. Detoxification is no longer a luxury. It's essential to living in the body you deserve.

## Self-Assessment

Do you have or have you experienced in the past six months . . .

☐ Fatigue, even when you get the coveted eight hours of sleep?

☐ Fatigue after exercising?

☐ Withdrawal symptoms when you stop eating foods like refined carbs, sugar, or caffeine, such as feeling jittery, shaky, irritable, and just not right? Or a heartbroken feeling like you are pining after a long-lost love?

☐ Achy joints?

☐ Frequent colds, particularly bronchitis and chest congestion in the winter?

☐ Ears that itch or tinnitus (ringing in the ears)?

☐ Hives, rashes, or dry skin?

☐ Dark circles or bags under your eyes? Itchy eyes or increased mucus in your eyes when you wake up in the morning?

☐ Brain fog and/or poor memory?

☐ Weight loss, but then you hit a plateau or regain it?

☐ A puffy-looking face, like you're retaining fluid?

☐ Difficulty recovering from a major stress, such as a surgery?

☐ Mood swings, including depression, anxiety, and/or irritability?

☐ Tummy troubles, such as gas, bloating, nausea, burping, or heartburn?

☐ Breath so bad you are constantly rummaging around in your purse for a mint?

### Interpret Your Results

- **If you have five or more of these symptoms,** you need at least a three-day Toxin Free reset.

- **If you have fewer than five of these symptoms or are unsure,** you could have a lower burden than others. But you aren't off the hook! I recommend a detox anyway. Done correctly, it has no negative repercussions and can only make you feel even better.

---

### From Dr. Sara's Case Files: Ginny, Age Fifty-Five

---

- *Lost 21 pounds on the Hormone Reset Diet.*
- *Learned that environmental toxins are a common cause of blood sugar problems and weight gain.*
- *"I have more energy and am better able to handle my extremely stressful job. My energy and sleeping [have] vastly improved. My blood sugar is much better controlled. Before, my fasting blood sugar was 96 to 107 and my postprandials were usually around 130 mg/dL [or higher]. I thought that going off sugar would make me a crazy-eating machine. Now, my fasting blood sugar is 82 to 90, and my postprandials are 86 to 100. I have PCOS, and this is a fabulous outcome. I wasn't perfect all the time, but I didn't beat myself up about that. My edema in my legs [and] feet is gone. My facial hair growth has slowed dramatically."*

- *Lost 8 inches overall (arms, bust, waist, hips, thighs).*
- *"The realization finally hit me that unlike other 'diet' plans where everything is prescribed by limits and/or exacting quantities, the concept about really HONORING what my body is telling is the key. In the old days, if I could eat four slices a day as my top limit, by golly, I was going to make sure I got it. Now, I listen!"*

## The Science Behind Toxin Free

You are confronted with an astounding number of toxins each day, including pesticides, herbicides, genetically modified foods, and about six different synthetic hormones in meat. Toxins are lurking in the fire-retardant materials in couches, the linings of tuna fish cans, face creams, prescription drugs, processed foods, as heavy metals in the environment and your lipstick, even the air you breathe. The list goes on.

The molecular sex in your body—that is, the interaction between a hormone in charge of your metabolism and its receptor—is disrupted by toxins.

Ultimately, toxins make you numb to insulin and leptin, and they are linked to the development of blood sugar issues, lowered immunity, increased inflammation, stroke, and a vulnerability to autoimmune disorders.[2] One study showed that a particular type of persistent organic pollutant (POP)—a class called organochloride pesticides—is linked to weight gain of 9.5 pounds over fifty years when you have high concentrations compared with people with the lowest concentrations.[3] Your risk of weight gain and disease from exposure to toxins may be woefully underestimated. There is scientific evidence of a link between plastic-associated synthetic chemicals and heart disease, and the proof that they make you fat and insulin resistant is stronger. Taken together, the constellation of problems warrants application of the precautionary principle: assume these toxins are guilty until proven innocent.

A survey by the Centers for Disease Control and Prevention demonstrated that 93 percent of the population has measurable levels of bisphenol A (BPA), a chemical that disrupts your estrogen, thyroid, and androgen hormones and is found in store receipts and canned foods. Endocrine disruptors have been shown to interfere with the production, transportation, and metabolism of most hormones.

We detox to rid our bodies of the inevitable buildup of toxins that happens in modern life. A detox is the perfect antidote for resetting your entire system so you can move forward with lightness and clarity. Daily exposure to environmental toxins can have a major impact on your health and can lead to becoming overweight. This fact makes me feel that the term "endocrine disruptors" doesn't go far enough. Xenobiotics, a term that refers to chemical compounds that are foreign to an organism, also seems insufficient. We should call them metabolic blockers, since they block your metabolism *and* your endocrine system from performing their divine functions. I also call them party crashers, because they were not designed by your Maker to be in on the awesome party happening in your body, mind, and soul.

Detoxing is crucial for your long-term health. It boosts metabolism, helps remove estrogen-disrupting chemicals, improves thyroid functioning, and rids the body of extra toxins released in the bloodstream when you lose weight. Not to mention that you'll feel clear, clean, and energetic. What have you got to lose?

## Metabolism Blockers May Make You Fat

In the Toxin Free reset, the focus is on reducing exposure to and removing synthetic chemicals that block your metabolism and may make you fat. There are three main classes of metabolism blockers that cause undesirable hormone effects by adversely impacting your androgen, estrogen, and thyroid systems. They act by various mechanisms, such as fooling the body into an exaggerated response, blocking hormone receptors, slowing down or speeding up enzymes that convert one hormone into another, and causing liver damage (and raising liver enzyme levels, as measured in a simple blood test).

*Androgen disruptors.* Metabolism blockers that impact androgens include bisphenol A, phthalates, and mycotoxins.[4] In general, androgen disruptors raise testosterone in women and lower testosterone in men. For instance, adolescent girls with higher levels of BPA are more likely to be diagnosed with polycystic ovary syndrome, and BPA levels correlate significantly with testosterone levels.[5] Additionally, phthalates and some mycotoxins, such as ochratoxin A, change aromatase, the enzyme that converts testosterone into estrogen.[6]

*Estrogen disruptors.* There are more than seven hundred synthetic chemicals that mimic estrogen in a toxic way, and their prevalence in our environment is on the rise. These toxins, found in an array of items from receipts to canned foods and from plastics to pesticides, have now been linked with early puberty, female infertility, ovulation, miscarriage, endometriosis, male infertility, obesity, diabetes, and an increase in certain cancers.[7]

*Thyroid disruptors.* As our exposure to endocrine disruptors has increased, so has the incidence of thyroid disease in the United States, particularly for thyroid cancer and thyroid autoimmune disease.[8] People who showed the highest 20 percent of exposure to environmental toxins also experienced up to 10 percent more thyroid function impairment than those with the 20 percent lowest exposure.[9] The most common exposure to thyroid disruptors is flame retardants, and the worst offender is your home and office furniture.

*Mixed hormone disruptors.* Some metabolic blockers, such as bisphenol A (BPA), promote weight gain via multiple hormone pathways. BPA disrupts estrogen, thyroid, androgen, adiponectin, leptin, and ghrelin function in the human body.[10] The most common exposures include handling receipts and eating food from BPA-lined cans.

Okay, we know these toxins are bad. So, how do we get rid of them? You may be as surprised as I was to learn that eating food containing olestra has been shown to reduce your toxic load of endocrine disruptors, specifically polychlorinated biphenyls (PCBs, used as a fluid coolant in electrical systems) and dichloro-diphenyldichloroethylene (DDE, a pesticide and reproductive toxin responsible for the decline of the bald eagle).[11] Even if eating these items seems to work, my common sense tells me there must be a better way. And there is: Look no further than your trusty organ the liver, which is your body's natural filter, designed to purify the blood and remove toxins.

Your liver does this in two phases that my friend Dr. Holly Lucille calls garbage generation (phase one) and garbage collection (phase two). In phase one, your liver takes toxins like BPA out of your blood and converts them into molecules known as metabolites. In phase two, your liver sends the toxic metabolites to be removed from the body in your urine or stool. In other words, you take out the garbage, like I do every Sunday night at my home.

Unfortunately, most of us have a problem with both phases. From stress and constant exposure to toxins, you may have an overactive phase one and create too much garbage—some of which is worse than the original toxin itself. Then, to make matters worse, you forget to collect the garbage by neglecting your body's need for detox. It keeps piling up, as if the garbage collectors were on strike. The result is that your liver isn't doing its job of detoxification, which can lead to all sorts of symptoms, such as hives, rashes, itchy eyes, anxiety, and weight gain. By increasing your intake of key minerals, fiber, and other nutrients, you can strengthen the garbage collection and removal capacity of the liver.

## MITO-WHAT?

You might remember the word from your high school science class: mitochondria. As a cell's utility company, mitochondria generate chemical energy. Think of how you plug in your smartphone to charge it. Similarly, your mitochondria charge your cells so they can do their jobs. Why should you care? When not taken care of, mitochondria can't charge your cells and they form free radicals, which can lead to all sorts of problems, from fatigue to multiple sclerosis to cancer.

The moral of the story is mind your mitochondria before the charge stops working. Since xenobiotics, drugs, and pollution can lead to their decay, take a careful look at the toxins you are letting into your body. Do what you can to reduce exposure and boost health: exercise and restrict refined carbohydrates. Amp up the fresh air, clean proteins, and veggies. Supplement with a multivitamin, ubiquinal, N-acetylcysteine, resveratrol, and magnesium. When you take good care of your mito-chondria, you empower your body to power your life.

## BUYER BEWARE: INVESTIGATE YOUR BEAUTY PRODUCTS

Know what lurks in your beauty products, because many contain some of the 700 known xenoestrogens or even estrogen itself. What you don't know can make you fat, cranky, foggy, and maybe even cancerous. Sadly, your quest for youthful looks may have the opposite effect, causing excess estrogen to enter your body through your moisturizer or shampoo.

*Here are a few actions you can take to avoid the most common fake estrogens that mimic the action of estrogen in the body and are often found in your cosmetics.*

## Avoid Parabens

*Parabens are a fake estrogen preservative used in about 85 percent of lotions and lipsticks, and they're linked to endocrine and developmental problems. You find them in many skin creams. In its studies, the Centers for Disease Control and Prevention has found parabens in all Americans surveyed, which confirms that they are ubiquitously stored in the body. While the evidence is not yet firm that parabens actually cause cancer, apply the precautionary principle.*

### Your Hormone Reset Solution

*When you can, buy paraben-free products, such as Aveda, Dr. Hauschka, Josie Maran Cosmetics, and Origins. Do your research before you buy.*

## Avoid Phthalates

*Phthalates, another form of xenoestrogen (fake estrogen), are added to shampoos, deodorants, body washes, hair gels, hair sprays, and nail polishes for fragrance. Phthalates have been found to cause birth defects in male fetuses. One form of phthalate, called diethylhexyl phthalate (DEHP), is allowed by the FDA in foods that mainly contain water. Scary.*

### Your Hormone Reset Solution

*One of the best ways to avoid phthalates is to check labels and vote for phthalate-free beauty products with your dollars. Phthalates are known as "everywhere chemicals" because they are so commonly used, not just in beauty products but in most plastics we use daily. Another way to reduce your exposure is to avoid microwaving your food in plastic containers.*

**Avoid Sodium Lauryl Sulfate**

*Here's yet another fake estrogen used commonly in soaps, tooth-pastes, and shampoos. There is some concern that exposure may be linked to breast cancer and also to a drop in male fertility.*

**Your Hormone Reset Solution**

*Once again, check labels. Use organic soaps, toothpastes, and sham-poos. For more information, check out the Environmental Working Group's Skin Deep database of sixty-eight thousand cosmetics.*

---

# Get Your Micronutrients

When it comes to detoxing, my task with patients is to find the obsta-cles to their detoxification and remove them. Most of my patients get very focused on the macronutrients (relative quantities of protein, fat, carbohydrates) yet few understand the role of micronutrients, such as vitamins, amino acids, polysaccharides, and minerals. In this reset, I want to shine the love lights on minerals. Plain and simple, minerals detoxify you, and you probably are running low on many of them. They are instrumental to 95 percent of the delicate biochemistry in the body, and if you've been a carb addict for years, you are probably deficient in minerals.

You've already heard me talk about magnesium in chapter 2 (see page 37), and now I want to get serious about sulfur, another crucial mineral to your detoxification and health.[12] My friend David Wolfe calls sulfur the "world's best cosmetic" because it's fundamental to the health of your hair, skin, and nails. My colleague Dr. Stephanie Seneff, senior scientist at MIT and pioneer in sulfur research, says that sulfur deficiency is far more pervasive than most people realize, and the majority of conventional physicians seem unaware of the pivotal role played by sulfur in proper insulin function.

When it comes to detoxification, sulfur relieves inflammation and helps to turn on the fat-burning machine. Where do you find it? Dietary proteins, including fish, organic and/or pastured beef and poultry, coconut and olive oils, arugula, bee pollen, hemp, broccoli, Brussels sprouts, blue-green algae, kale, pumpkin seeds, radishes, spirulina, and watercress.

Are you short on sulfur? A deficiency is common and heralded by obesity, heart disease, Alzheimer's disease, chronic fatigue, acne, arthritis, brittle hair and nails, gastrointestinal challenges, immune system dysfunction, lingering muscle injuries, memory loss, rashes, scar tissue, and slow wound healing.

Sulfur isn't the only need-to-know mineral. Selenium, copper, and zinc are important for your thyroid, and the copper-to-zinc ratios must be kept in order. Taking a high-potency multivitamin keeps the ratio in check. Sea salt contains important minerals too, such as trace amounts of calcium, potassium, magnesium, zinc, and iron.[13]

You also need to fill in the nutritional gaps related to amino acids, the building blocks of protein. Here are a few favorites:

- *Glutathione* is a powerful antioxidant that your body produces to detox free radicals. I think of it as your antirust protector.

- *N-acetylcysteine* is the precursor of glutathione (see the Supplements section, page 210).

## Toxin Free: The Three-Day Reset for Testosterone and Other Hormones

Our final reset augments the previous six food-based resets by addressing environmental factors that may make you fat and upgrading your body's own detoxification pathways. In addition to being mindful about what you put into your body, let's address what you put onto your body. The skin absorbs many environmental toxins and sometimes makes them even worse once inside. Over the next three days, you'll swap the metabolic blockers for natural products, replace your missing minerals and other nutrients, and upgrade your liver and gut function.

## TOXIN FREE RULES: DO THESE EACH DAY

In the Toxin Free reset, you are integrating the previous six resets and deepening detoxification by replacing two meals with a clean protein shake.

1. **Be wary of skin products.** When you wake up in the morning, become increasingly aware of what you put on your skin and mucosal membranes such as your mouth. Start with your first action. If you're like me, you scrape your tongue and brush your teeth after arising from bed. Make sure the first product(s) you apply are free of metabolic blockers, such as organic toothpaste or deodorant, natural shampoos and conditioners, biodynamic soap or lotions. (See Resources for recommended brands.)

2. **Up your intake of alkaline-forming foods.** An easy way to do this is to start your morning with a hot cup of water with lemon, followed by a green shake for breakfast. Aim for two to three servings of greens each day.

3. **Continue to eat one pound or more of vegetables every day.** Prepare your pound accordingly: half lightly cooked, half raw. (Note: if you have thyroid issues, lightly cook all your veggies.) Cruciferous vegetables boost both phases of liver detoxification—make sure to consume cabbage, broccoli, and Brussels sprouts. Add vegetables to your shakes to keep volume high. Alliums such as onions and scallions will boost Phase II liver detoxification.

4. **Keep up your fiber consumption of 35 to 45 grams per day.** If you're gut is feeling fine (no gas or bloating), you can try higher amounts. Fiber helps to bind metabolic blockers.

5. **Add seeds and spices to your cooking.** Caraway and dill seeds improve Phase I of liver detoxification (garbage generation), and curcumin (turmeric), rosemary, thyme, and oregano help Phase II.

6. **Make sure your food containers are safe** by using glass and stainless steel. Avoid storing or cooking food in plastic containers.

7. **Get outside.** I was shocked to learn from the Environmental Protection Agency that the air we breathe inside the home could be up to five times more polluted than the air outside. During the Toxin Free reset, consider getting outside more, opening more windows in your home, running a HEPA filter, putting encasements on your pillows and mattresses, and replacing toxic home cleaning products. If that feels too ambitious, focus on a brisk walk outside after a meal for fifteen to twenty minutes, and get rid of one or two cleaning products. Household cleaning products contain more than 17,000 chemicals, and only a fraction have been tested for their effects on human health. Use white vinegar, herbs, borax, olive oil, and lemon juice as safer ingredients for cleaning, and see Resources for recommended recipes.

## SAMPLE MENU

On the following page is a suggested menu for resetting your estrogen, insulin, leptin, testosterone, and thyroid. For nutritional data, check out the Notes section.[14]

### WATER FILTERS: THE LOWDOWN

*It's important to drink extra water during the Toxin Free reset to flush out impurities. But what if the water itself is toxic? Water can contain any number of scary contaminants, including lead, fluoride, chlorine, arsenic, nitrates, sulfates, herbicides, pesticides, bacteria,*

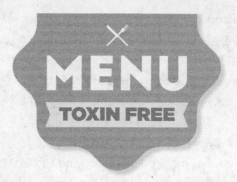

## MENU
### TOXIN FREE

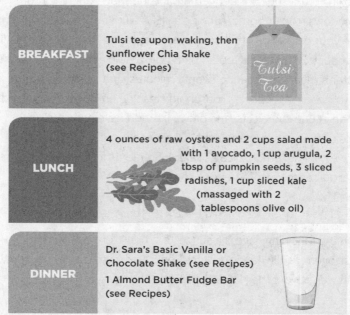

**BREAKFAST**

Tulsi tea upon waking, then Sunflower Chia Shake (see Recipes)

**LUNCH**

4 ounces of raw oysters and 2 cups salad made with 1 avocado, 1 cup arugula, 2 tbsp of pumpkin seeds, 3 sliced radishes, 1 cup sliced kale (massaged with 2 tablespoons olive oil)

**DINNER**

Dr. Sara's Basic Vanilla or Chocolate Shake (see Recipes) 1 Almond Butter Fudge Bar (see Recipes)

*and other microorganisms like parasites. So, the first step to getting a water filter is testing the tap water in your home.*

*Assessing for a range of common contaminants can cost more than one hundred dollars, but the investment is worthwhile because it can help you identify the best system for your water. When you test, keep an eye especially on the two most common contaminants: chlorine* and lead. The Environmental Protection Agency estimates that 20 percent of lead exposure comes from water.

Once you know what you are dealing with, you might want to consider purchasing a home water purifying system, like I did. These systems vary greatly in effectiveness and cost. Here's a small sampling:

- **Alkaline water filters.** Proponents claim that alkaline water neutralizes acid in the blood and fights free radicals. But I am wary about these systems, which often cost thousands of dollars.

- **Carbon filters.** This method uses activated carbon to absorb impurities in your water. They vary greatly; some just remove chlorine, while others remove a wider variety of contaminants. I use a carbon filter that I purchased online for less than thirty dollars. I think these inexpensive carbon filters are the way to go to keep your water clean and your detox in full gear.

- **Reverse osmosis systems.** This method pushes water through a membrane that blocks certain particles. These sometimes contain carbon filters, and the best option appears to be the combination.

For more details, visit the Environmental Working Group's Water Filter Buying Guide.[15]

### WHAT TO EXPECT WHEN YOU'RE . . . DETOXING

Toxin Free is a big change for your system, which is accustomed to brand-name toothpaste, shampoo, and plastics. The first day or so you might notice symptoms that are familiar from some of your past resets. Just stay with it, observing the discomfort instead of getting wrapped up in it. Know that you are doing this for a good reason. If you feel discouraged or tempted, rely on a buddy system, write in your journal, or ask for divine help.

*Symptoms during your detox might include:*
- *mood swings*
- *irritability*
- *restlessness*
- *nightmares*
- *acne*
- *headaches*

---

# Supplements

Supplements can put you on the detox fast track by helping you eliminate toxic chemicals that might be building up in your body. There is a dizzying array of detox products on the market that claim to restore your body's balance. Many of the following supplements I've discussed in previous resets, but they are serving double duty when you are Toxin Free. One of the most important is N-acetylcysteine, but keep up your supplementation with fiber and a daily multivitamin too!

- *N-acetylcysteine (NAC).* NAC is derived from the amino acid l-cysteine. (Amino acids are building blocks of proteins.) NAC has been used for many years in medicine for detoxification of the liver, such as in people who get too much acetaminophen (Tylenol). I recently found that my mercury and lead levels are high, so I take NAC to reduce my levels of these toxic metals. Overall, NAC is a great supplement to support your detoxification. I recommend 600 mg once or twice per day.

- *A high-potency multivitamin.* This will improve the enzyme-dependent detoxification pathways.

# Cell to Soul Practice

News flash: your thought patterns just might be contributing to your overall toxic burden. If you are anything like me, your mind is going a mile a minute. Sometimes you feel like you can't have a clear thought. Some of this is hormonal; I've addressed brain fog, fatigue, depression, and anxiety at length in my previous book, *The Hormone Cure*. Some of my unhelpful (to put it nicely) thoughts are the result of the ingrained patterns I've gathered over decades. In yoga, these thought patterns are called samskaras. Just like the grooves of a record that get deeper and deeper the more you play it, the thoughts in the mind get more ingrained the more they are repeated. There is a scientific backing for this, called neuroplasticity. This is why negative thought patterns are difficult to release and insidious. Over time, they can hijack your heart and mind without you even realizing it.

It's time to detoxify your mind. It takes some work, because sometimes toxic thoughts happen in an instant: one tiny word can trigger a series of thoughts and emotions . . . and off you go.

As a woman of science, I always like to look for a process. That's why I challenge you to apply the Socratic method to your thoughts—and then write out what you discover. Let's say you are a worrier. The first step is noticing each worried thought. This simple act alone will make you keenly aware of how much time and energy you dedicate to worrying. Once you are able to notice these worries, start to ask questions. For example, if you have a minor symptom like a cough that you're convinced is lung cancer, try applying Socratic questioning instead of getting carried away with worried thoughts. *What is the evidence for this? What are the odds of this happening? Am I being fully objective?* Over time, you'll see more clearly how your thoughts can be counterproductive. Sometimes I like to talk to my thoughts, telling them they are irrational, made up, or just ridiculous. Sometimes I get mad at my thoughts for trying to control me. But most of the time I try to replace them with positive ones.

Another possibility is taking a particular worry to its utmost conclusion and asking yourself what's the worst that can happen if one of your worries comes true. Of course that's not for everyone. Some of us might just worry more.

When we let go of something—negative feelings, an old hurt or wound, something we really needed to say—we feel lighter too. Whether or not you're trying to lose weight, discharging heavy emotions and petty annoyances leaves you with a lightness. It feels like lifting a weight off your shoulders.

Norman Vincent Peale, author of *The Power of Positive Thinking*, suggested a way of examining your negative emotions. For twenty-four hours, every time you feel frustrated or irritated, write it down—no matter how petty or minor the annoyance. At the end of twenty-four hours, review the list. Does it give you insight into what you need to let go of?

In your journal, write down your negative thought and then your positive counterstatement. Over time, you'll be able to detox your mind, releasing unnecessary fear and worry. And while you are at it, use that very same journal each night to write down things that went well or things you feel grateful for in your life. Science shows that this process, done repeatedly, will bring you more happiness through simply acknowledging the positive.

## Exercise

Yoga encompasses the belief that we all have an inner fire that needs to be stoked for proper digestion and detoxification. To this end, yoga has many *kriyas*, or cleansing practices, designed to clear the physical and subtle bodies. I love *agni sara*, a *kriya* that burns up impurities in the energy bodies. It's an advanced practice that is considered foundational for many yogis: *agni* means "fire," and *sara* means "essence." In this practice, you contract the muscles from the floor of your pelvis to your diaphragm while emptying out your breath. The act of creating heat in the internal organs boosts circulation, improves elimination, and releases toxins. These aren't the only benefits. Working with the core also helps you connect with your center, bring awareness to your breath, and get in touch with your emotions.

Here's how to do it:

1. Stand in a comfortable position with your feet spread 3 feet apart and your knees bent at 90-degree angles (known as "horse stance").

2. Bring your hands to your thighs, coming into a slight squat while keeping your back erect, not rounded.

3. Exhale completely. Holding the breath out, contract your pelvic floor and abdomen, "sucking" your belly in and up. The whole front of your body should be contracted and the breath should be emptied out. Pump the diaphragm in and out five times, while still not breathing, keeping all breath out.

4. After the final pump, take a deep inhale and release the contraction.

5. Continue with these exhalations and inhalations, making them as smooth and steady as you can.

6. Repeat the sequence five times, and gradually build up to thirty repetitions.

## Test Yourself

Your body is designed to detoxify, but sometimes there are roadblocks. In my first book, *The Hormone Cure,* I talked about the importance of organ reserve—the capacity of an organ, such as your liver, thyroid, or adrenal glands, to function beyond its baseline needs. When it comes to detoxification, the most important organs on your team are your liver, gut, skin, kidneys, fat, and lungs. You can detoxify your lungs with exercise, sweating, and breathing practices. Moreover, it's worthwhile to test your liver in a simple blood test (performed by most doctors in an annual checkup) called alanine aminotransferase (ALT). The ALT level in your blood is primarily produced in the liver, as well as in lesser amounts in the heart, muscles, kidneys, and pancreas. The ALT level indicates whether the liver is diseased or injured.

## Notes from Hormone Resetters

"I completed my chemo, radiation, and Herceptin treatment for breast cancer. I had gained weight and lost many other things, my self-esteem and my not-so-bad-looking body and my beautiful hair. My friend recommended your program, and it worked for her! I was ready to look and feel better. Needless to say, I feel great and lost 12 pounds in a delightful way, and I even did it while on vacation!" —*Rhona*

"My main reason for going on the [program] was to eliminate unnecessary toxins in my body. In the middle, I experienced serenity and lots of energy. I learned much more than I expected to learn from the program, and Dr. Gottfried does an amazing job in explaining not only what you need to do, but why, and she uses the latest information available today from the best science out there. It is a great learning experience, and you will feel great afterwards." —*Mark*

# Final Word

*Courage transforms fear.* I encourage you to use this as a sacred time to clear off the dust and discover how courageous you can be toward yourself. Take an inventory of your fears. Release your fears along with the toxins. Start anew from the powerful, strong center within—a resource you can always count on, no matter what is happening in the external world. Cross the bridge from fear with courage and reach toward your deepest and most heartfelt dreams.

Remember to invite the Divine into your life by setting up a regular practice of prayer—whether it's attending church, walking in the woods or near the ocean, or just spending quiet time clearing your mind each day.

I suspect you'll be surprised at how many environmental toxins and synthetic chemicals we expose ourselves to each day. Many of these products are metabolism blockers. It's important to identify the worst culprits, reduce your exposure, and replace them with healthier alternatives.

Good luck with the Toxin Free reset. I've seen profound results when it's approached with an open heart and mind. When you give yourself permission to release ingrained habits that don't serve you anymore, integrate what you've learned, and honor what is unique for your body, my hunch is that you just might find a profound and renewed connection to your life.

# PART THREE

# Reentry and Beyond

# CHAPTER 10

# Reentry

Day 22

Congratulations. You've completed a major step in reclaiming your body and your health. At times, it hasn't been easy. But you did it! After twenty-one days, you are recalibrated, pure, and clean. Before we start reintroducing foods we've eliminated, let's reflect a moment. Take a deep breath, draw in the positive, and revel in all you've accomplished. If nothing else, the Hormone Reset Diet shows you that you can get better, smarter, and wiser with age when you develop certain practices that support, rather than diminish, your long-term health.

Now what? Like an astronaut coming back to earth after a successful mission, you can't just haphazardly step out and hope for the best. You've reset your hormones, and we need to protect your new habits. Accordingly, you need to plan carefully for your reentry into the orbit of real life.

I know you can see that the end is near, and you may be tempted to jump ahead and start eating a few "challenge foods" before your body is ready. I strongly urge you to be patient with Reentry, which starts on Day 22 and lasts as long as you need to collect data and integrate the information. (You may need to take more time. Most people add back three foods only between Days 22 to 30, but duration varies depending on the foods you reintroduce). During this time, you will add back one food at a time and see how your body reacts for three full days. It may just be the most important part of the Hormone Reset. Why? Because you are collecting very important data about your body that will continue to guide your personal food code for months and years to come.

## Why Reentry?

You've removed the most allergenic foods and metabolic blockers that make your immune system overreact. You have a sacred opportunity, hard earned, to stay in close contact with the innate wisdom of your body and to learn intimately how it responds to food.

Just as you took three days to reset each hormone and remove the worst food culprits, we will reintroduce only one reset food at a time—and closely observe your response. When you do this, you will cultivate a whole new level of body awareness. Attune to the wisdom of your body. Ultimately, your goal is to act in a way that creates a positive outcome.

## Your Personal Food Code

The first step in Reentry is creating a personal food code, which states in written form your personal commitment when it comes to food and nourishment.

When you write things down, you will be able to track subtle and tiny adjustments that your body makes in response to food. Remember that you can edit your personal food code during the Reentry phase. It's a living document that will shift according to your internal and external demands.

In drafting your personal food code, consider how you want to be in relationship to food and health. This is your chance to dream big! The idea is to create your boundaries around food and to live deliberately and aligned with the food guidelines that you've established for yourself.

Your personal food code can be short or long. Use bullet points. Call it something that speaks to you: "Manifesto," "Feminesto," "Road Map." As author Dr. Rick Hanson advises, this could be a "handful of words, or dos and don'ts. Whatever its form, aim for language that is powerful and motivating, that makes sense to your head and touches your heart."[1] He goes on to suggest that it needn't be perfect to be of great value and that periodic revisions are highly encouraged.

### DR. SARA'S PERSONAL FOOD CODE

*This is my personal food code that I use as a touchstone for my meal plan. I offer it as an example for you to gain inspiration or to edit for yourself.*

- *Focus on awareness when it comes to food. Learn to do what's best for my body, cell to soul.*
- *Meditate every morning for thirty minutes.*
- *Approach the planning, shopping, chopping, cooking, and eating as a sadhana, a spiritual practice.*
- *Choose organic, non-GM, pastured, clean, and best-quality foods that are known to keep my blood sugar balanced. Eat more superfoods, and be mindful of the subtle energetics of the plant.*
- *Drink more filtered water.*
- *Write down all meals with portion sizes the night before, and stick to the plan the next day.*
- *Eat prior to parties and events where the food won't meet my food code or is unknown.*

- *Avoid dairy, gluten, sugar, and grains. (I'm intolerant.)*
- *Take three deep, lower-belly breaths, inhaling the aroma of the food, before taking the first bite.*
- *Listen attentively—specifically, put the fork down and chew (chew a lot!). Stop eating when I'm 70 percent full.*
- *Model healthy eating for my children and my community.*

———————

Keep revisiting, revising, and updating your food code over time so that it truly works for you. When you overindulge or eat foods that are best avoided, recalibrate. Record what helps you get back on track. Record what derails you. Keep refining so that your food code is like your code of ethics around food—your bottom line when it comes to creating your best health.

## Reactions to Reentry

It's essential that you continue to foster mind–body alignment as you progress through Reentry. In the ongoing dialogue between food and your body, you may learn in this phase exactly what foods must be eliminated from your long-term food plan. About ten years ago, when I first went through the elimination diet that became the Hormone Reset, I was very sad to learn that I can't tolerate gluten or dairy. Even more sadly, I found that I couldn't cheat at all. There is something very beautiful and solemn about listening to the will of your body, instead of imposing the will of your mind onto your body.

In my experience, there are three different mind-sets that happen during Reentry.

- *Easy Peasy.* Some people who go through Reentry add back one challenge food at a time, taking three days to listen to how the body responds, and they don't have any adverse reactions that signal intolerance. Minimal detective work is needed.

- *Let's Get This Going, Already.* Others get impatient and add back two foods at a time, such as cheese and grains. Then they gain weight or experience bloating and gas, but don't know which food was the trigger. They lost the benefit of the clean slate, since it's impossible to know which challenge food was the problem.

- *More Challenging than Expected.* Still others notice that they become addicted again when they reintroduce their challenge food, and they see the breakdown in their body awareness—the disconnect between mind and body as they add a food back into the matrix—especially sugar, or liquid sugar in the form of alcohol. Your body may send you the divine message that the challenge food isn't digesting well or you can't tolerate it, but your mind doesn't want to adjust. This situation requires the most detective work, curiosity, and body awareness.

In each situation, you can use key questions: *How is this food talking to me? What is it trying to teach me?* Normally the food–body conversation is one-way: *I need to eat X for dinner.* But it turns out the food–body conversation is two-directional. Listen closely, and you might be surprised at what you hear.

## Teach a Woman to Fish

The idea of reintroducing food after an elimination diet is not novel. The process of elimination and provocation is the gold standard when it comes to identifying allergenic foods. Yet for harried modern women, what is new is body awareness, plus a newfound ability to adjust and tweak in response to the subtle effects of food on the female body. This calibration of finer reactions allows you to personalize your food so it suits you best. Indeed, it is your path to personal power around food and weight, and it is the secret to staying lean and sustaining your progress.

Remember the Chinese proverb: give a man a fish and you feed him for a day; *teach a man to fish* and you feed him for a lifetime. Similarly, at this point in the program, it won't serve you for me to tell you what to do and for you to robotically go through the motions while ignoring the reactions of your body. That would be giving you the fish, but the female body is not one-size-fits-all. Your best food program is a complex mash-up of your biological age, stress, mind–body practices, life stage, genetics, metabolic rate, fitness level, and vulnerabilities and strengths.

Instead of simply receiving the fish, accept my invitation to evolve and become wiser about how food affects your body, hormones, and weight. Now that you have a clean slate, you're ready to learn to fish with the process of trial, tweak, and triumph. It will allow you to get in touch with your food truths, and very few people have this blessed chance to learn about how food talks to their biology. I revere this moment in time now that you've completed your Hormone Reset. I challenge you to hit the pause button and become completely present to it before you race back to business as usual.

Now that you've cleaned up your food, removed the most common food irritants, and broken your addictive patterns, another opportunity before you is to upgrade the nutrient density of the foods you choose to keep in your food plan. I encourage you to turn to the highest quality protein and vegetable sources to get the nutrient density you need.

## SUPERFOODS ARE YOUR ALLIES

*It's a bird. It's a plane. It's . . . superfoods! These foods are just as exciting as they sound: foods that are superconcentrated with nutrients and thought to boost the immune system, increase energy, and create balance in the body. You might have heard of them: cacao, maca,* raw hemp, sea vegetables, bee pollen, and medicinal mushrooms, to name a few.

These super allies, found at your local health food store, are said to lower your cholesterol, reduce your risk of cancer, and boost your mood.[2] What's the deal with the super magic of these superfoods? The superfoods are rich in the subtle energy and intelligence of the plant kingdom, the undefiled nutrients from the freshest possible sources that go directly from a farm to you. Here are my favorite superfoods:

- oysters
- wild-caught salmon
- turkey
- blueberries
- broccoli
- oranges
- tomatoes
- pumpkin
- greens such as kale, chard, and spinach
- green tea
- walnuts
- yogurt

## ANCESTRAL GUIDANCE

The functional medicine expert and acupuncturist Chris Kresser, one of the most articulate and thoughtful leaders in the Ancestral Health movement, taught me a lot about the Paleo diet, such as that all organisms are designed to adapt and survive in a particular environment. If the environment changes faster than the adaptation, there's a mismatch, which may lead to negative consequences. This is not just his synthesis but the fundamental rule of evolutionary biology. Therefore, there's a certain diet that humans are fairly well adapted to eat: fish, wild game, pastured and clean meat, vegetables, sweet potatoes, seeds, and nuts. About ten thousand years ago, the rise of agriculture introduced us to grains, legumes, alcohol, and dairy.

This explanation led to a major aha moment for me. I realized that some of us (myself included) aren't well adapted to these Johnny-come-lately foods. While some of us do fine with them, I'm intolerant. When I eat them, I damage my gut, become inflamed, and gain weight. Now that we are in Reentry, I'll ask you: How well adapted you are to consuming meat, grains, legumes, alcohol, and dairy?

---

## Reentry: The Three-Day Challenge

The time has come. You need to take the slow descent back into the atmosphere. Take a final check before all systems go. It's time to begin your Reentry, the essential piece of the puzzle in discovering your food intolerances and allergies.

### REENTRY RULES

You will be reintroducing one food at a time and observing your response for three days. Here are the steps for a smooth Reentry:

1. **Draft your personal food code in your journal.**

2. **Choose your challenge food**—the one you had the hardest time giving up or craved the most. Keep in mind what my friend JJ Virgin, author of *The Virgin Diet,* taught me: sometimes the hardest food to give up and the one you miss the most is the one that you're most reactive toward, either as a slow-down for your metabolism or as a food intolerance or allergy.

3. **Eat your challenge food at one meal,** beginning on Day 22. Eat the food again on Day 23 and Day 24—ideally at the same meal and only once per day.

4. **Trial, tweak, and triumph.** Watch your response to the food for three days, including the food–mood connection, what happens

in your gut (bloating, gas, bowel movements, gurgling), to your body (discomfort, aches and pains), and to your pulse. Use the techniques and measurements I've described throughout the book, including weight, blood sugar, pulse, and food-mood journaling.

5. **Once you have carefully taken stock of your reactions** over three days, pick the next challenge food to test during the second set of three days.

6. **For those of you who want to take the reintroduction more slowly,** that's fine. Just don't go more quickly. Some people need to be on an elimination diet longer to reap benefits like weight loss and improved blood sugar. There is no one-size-fits-all, but the most important priority is attuning to what is true for you.

7. **You don't need to reintroduce all foods.** For instance, I know that I can't eat dairy, grains, or sugar. In my case, I will first reintroduce berries on Day 22 and trial, tweak, and triumph. On Day 25, I might eat grass-fed beef. On Day 28, I may drink a small glass of wine. As previously mentioned, your length of reentry will vary depending on how many foods you reintroduce.

### SAMPLE MENU

As an example, the menu option on the following page includes what to eat when your challenge food is dairy. For nutritional data, check out the Notes section.[3]

---

**"CAN'T I JUST CONTINUE THE RESETS?"**

*This is one of the most common questions I get at this point in the program. The short answer is yes, you are welcome to continue the resets for longer if you love the way you feel and want to continue improving upon your results, but a better solution is to shift after twenty-one days to Reentry and to perform the Hormone Reset Diet*

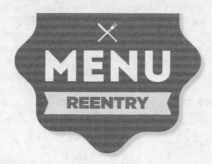

**BREAKFAST**

1 cup hot water with lemon and cayenne or herbal tea and Dr. Sara's Basic Vanilla or Chocolate Shake (see Recipes) with 2 tablespoons soaked chia seeds (alternative is Dr. Sara's Grain Free Pumpkin Porridge, see Recipes)

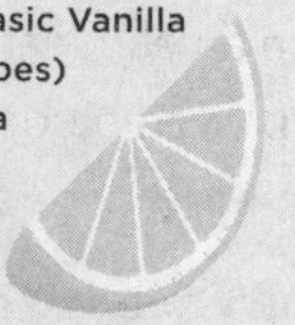

**LUNCH**

Before eating lunch, ¼ cup of coconut kefir
For lunch, eat 4 ounces white kidney beans, 1½ cups sliced chard (stems too!), plus ½ cup zucchini, all sautéed in 1 tablespoon organic, pastured ghee

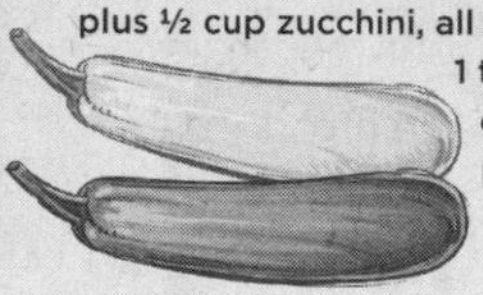

**DINNER**

4 to 6 ounces seared duck
6 ounces roasted sweet potatoes, red onions, and carrots
2 cups salad, such as Arugula Salad with Wild Mushrooms and Dairy-Free Brie (see Recipes)

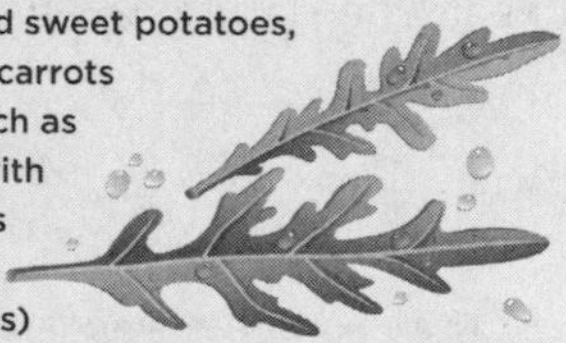

*once every three to six months. Note that you will continue to see results in the Reentry phase, but they may not be as dramatic as what you've experienced in the past twenty-one days.*

*However, it's important that you transition from resets to Reentry at some point in time. What you should not do is go straight from an extended period of resets to eating "normally" again. That's why I failed so many times before I discovered how the Hormone Reset works for me. The Reentry phase is critical for determining which foods are causing you to misfire, causing a reaction for you (allergic, intolerance, or hormonal/metabolic weight gain), and for giving your gut time to adjust to eating more of a challenge food again. If a food causes a reaction, keep it out of your food plan. Please allow at least six to fifteen days for the Reentry.*

---

## Reentry Tips and Tricks

- *Continue your daily rituals.* Whether it's a bath at night or hot water with lemon and cayenne in the morning, remember that these rituals help you systematize the resets that you are programming into your body and mind.

- *Take your shake.* Drink at least one shake per day and continue to get your pound of vegetables each day. (Yes, you can still do two shakes per day if you want to extend detoxification, but I don't recommend longer than ninety days total. There is such a thing as over-detoxing!)

- *Can I get a witness?* Focus on taking the role of an impartial observer. Instead of getting frustrated or feeling like you just reversed all the great work you've been doing or despairing that you can never eat this beloved food again, stop and take a deep breath. Now mentally remove yourself from your body and observe what's happening from the point of view of an (empathetic) stranger. It's never fun to feel bad or have your favorite things taken from you. But ultimately, this experience is a good thing because it's giving you more information about your body—information you can use to make healthy choices.

- *Be okay with your choices.* Some days your choices may mean indulging and dealing with the consequences. Other days you may choose to eliminate a substance from your diet completely. The choice is yours, and you are free to revise that choice at any time. But for today, just observe—and be kind to yourself.

- *Replete with red meat?* If after trying cleaner sources of protein and completing the Meatless reset you are convinced you really need red meat for energy, limit your intake to small amounts (4 to 6 ounces two or three times per week) of organic, grass-fed, or wild meat.

- *Measure and measure again.* Keep closer tabs on your measurements, particularly weight, blood sugar, hips, and waist. You've been measuring your weight once every three days during the resets. Now you want to weigh yourself daily, perform your other measurements, plus track your pulse, food–mood interactions, and other symptoms. It's easy to lose track. When you don't measure, you have to trust that eyeball estimate. My experience is that if I don't measure food portions, for example, I consistently overestimate what one cup looks like.

## Supplements

The most important supplement for you to take throughout Reentry and beyond is berberine. It's an anti-inflammatory! It's an antioxidant! It's an insulin sensitizer! Berberine lowers blood sugar as effectively as metformin, a common prescription used for women with polycystic ovary disease and diabetes, and that may come in handy during Reentry.[4] Found in the roots and barks of certain herbs, berberine helps treat or prevent fungal, parasitic, or bacterial infections.[5] I recommend 500 to 1,000 milligrams two to three times per day.

## Cell to Soul Practice

As a kid, I used to visit my father's family in Minnesota. Our relatives there, who were originally from Finland, all seemed to have dry saunas. We would hang out in the sauna as a family and then take a dip in a nearby icy lake. We kept alternating hot and cold because it felt so invigorating. Little did I know that this is one of the detoxifying techniques known as hydrotherapy. Hydrotherapy augments your body's natural detoxification. You can also replicate this technique in your shower: two minutes of hot water running over your body followed by two minutes of cold water. Try two to three cycles and see how you feel.

If your shower isn't doing it for you, try a local gym with a dry sauna, do a Google search for an infrared sauna near your home, or try a cryosauna, which uses the principle of "cold thermogenesis" to reduce inflammation, burn fat, and help reset your metabolic hormones.

## Exercise

My current obsession is to do plank pose for sixty seconds twice per day! There are a lot of benefits: confidence, core, back and arm strength, and more. It returns you to your center. I promise you big results for a tiny amount of time.

### CLEAN PROTEIN SOURCES AND HOW MUCH YOU MAY NEED

During Reentry, it's important that you get enough protein. Aim for 75 to 125 grams per day, depending upon your level of activity and weight. Some of the best protein sources and amounts for the average-weight woman are on the following chart.

# Eat More Clean Protein

| Food | Serving Size | Protein (grams) |
|------|--------------|-----------------|
| Oysters | 4 ounces (about 3 to 5 oysters, depending on size) | 24 |
| Salmon | 4 ounces | 28 |
| Halibut | 4 ounces | 30 |
| Eggs | 2 whole | 14 |
| Eggs | 2 whole plus 2 whites | 21 |
| Grass-fed ground beef | 4 ounces | 26 |
| Grass-fed filet mignon | 4 ounces | 24 |
| Duck | 4 ounces | 28 |
| Chicken breast | 4 ounces | 33–36 |
| Turkey | 4 ounces | 32 |
| Yogurt, plain, full fat | 4 ounces | 4 |
| Black beans | 4 ounces | 8 |
| Lentils | 4 ounces | 12 |
| Almonds | 1 ounce | 6 |
| Cashews | 1 ounce | 5 |
| Sunflower seeds | 1 ounce | 6 |
| Pumpkin seeds | 1 ounce | 7 |

## Test Yourself

Testing your pulse gives you valuable information about how you are responding to what you are ingesting. Perform the following three steps:

1. Before you eat one of your challenge foods, take your pulse when you are at rest.

2. Eat your challenge food.

3. Wait ten minutes, and check your pulse again. If your pulse has increased more than ten beats per minute, that suggests a reaction.

Please note that you may experience delayed reactions, such as itchy skin, rashes, or some of the other allergic responses, which can take three to four days to occur.

---

### From Dr. Sara's Case Files: Sylvie, Age Fifty-Three

- *Lost 18 pounds, 4 inches off her waist, and 4 inches off her hips.*
- *"I've determined that I'm a sugar addict and must not include it in my diet. Looks like I can't enjoy any more of those cakes and cupcakes I love to make."*
- *Blood sugar is down 25 points.*
- *"Had my first cup of coffee this morning and hate to say it didn't taste as it did" pre–Hormone Reset.*

---

## Notes from Hormone Resetters

"I'm following all of the things I learned. My weight eventually dropped to 115 pounds [total of 33 pounds lost—9 pounds in the first hormone reset]. I fluctuate a bit but after the good quality of life achieved from paying attention to my body, I am committed to this lifestyle." —*Tammy*

"Before I started, I was at my wits' end, trying to lose weight. I would follow diets carefully, but have very limited results. I exercised, but the scale still wouldn't budge. Now, I've learned some of the science behind why it was so hard to lose weight.

I had outgrown my fat pants and was rather hopeless. Despite what I thought was a healthy lifestyle, I felt like I was bound to be fat forever. Now, I feel like I have hope. I know that weight loss isn't just about calories in versus calories out. I better understand how to take care of my body and use food to nourish myself, not comfort myself. Which is now much easier since I have shed my 'sugar shackles'!" —*Linda*

"My blood sugar has dropped dramatically! I was at 118 a week before the Hormone Reset started. That freaked me out! So, no more sugar since then. Today my blood sugar was 86! Yippee! I had two grandparents that were diabetic, and my brother is diabetic (all type 2) . . . so I'm stopping that train right now. It was time to take my head out of the sand and look at some real numbers, and your [program] got me on the right track." —*Christy*

## Final Word

The final word for Reentry is "balance." On this journey, you've taken yourself to an extreme. You've spent time, money, brainpower, and internal resources in order to complete the twenty-one-day challenge. As you embrace Reentry, I want you to think of that pendulum swinging back to the center. My hope is that you don't feel like you are deprived or missing out, while at the same time you don't binge on sugar and alcohol. Balance. It's what makes us shine and become our best selves.

Take a look at all the things that help you feel balanced. Taking a five-minute break every hour? Saying "probably not" to another school volunteer opportunity? Then look at things that make you feel imbalanced. Overscheduling? Checking your smartphone constantly? Just like each person will have her own experience of Reentry, each person has her own definition of balance. It depends on your personality, life circumstances, and environment. What does balance mean to you?

The Reentry period is a good time to remember to practice the "Serenity Prayer" written originally by theologian Reinhold Niebuhr and adopted by twelve-step programs: God, grant me the serenity to accept the things I cannot change, the courage to change the things I can, and the wisdom to know the difference.

# CHAPTER 11

# Sustenance

I want to honor you for the extraordinary effort you've put into your Hormone Reset. I applaud your commitment, and I trust that it's paid off in terms of weight loss, inches lost, and glowing skin. If you are like my patients, your hormone problems are vastly better, and you have a glorious sense of feeling energetic and well rested. You've forged your own path and had inevitable breakthroughs with your unique biology.

Now that you've completed your Hormone Reset, it's time for the final, and perhaps most important, step of sustained weight loss: the continuation of a new way of eating. Most diets fail because people eat "clean" for a short time and then rebound to their old habits of either eating the wrong foods or eating too much food—or both. In order to sustain your weight loss and other benefits, we're going to change that.

In this chapter, we will review and refine your progress, self-awareness, and momentum so that you stay lean. As with the seven hormonal resets and the Reentry phase of your Hormone Reset, Sustenance is not about calorie restriction or weird juices. It's about defining and instituting a scientifically proven approach to staying on the path. This kind of sustenance might be a paradigm shift but one that will nourish you rather than deplete you. Sustenance will make you feel alive, instead of lethargic, grateful instead of resentful, hopeful instead of disheartened.

Now that you've reset your system and discovered your new baseline, you have new taste buds that are hungry for nutrient-dense food and a new set of receptors for the seven hormones of metabolism. Plus you're a fat-burning machine.

It's time to learn how to sustain your Hormone Reset habits. You have all the information you need. Your future is here. It's time to embrace it.

## Your Reboot

You know how your computer gets locked up occasionally and you have to restart it to get it operating smoothly again? That's what it's like when you shift to the last phase of your Hormone Reset: a reboot of your system. You are crossing a new threshold in your body. Your body is clean and tuned, your gut has been repaired, your mitochondria are working smoothly, your immune system is happy, and you've quelled the inflammation that makes you fat. Now what do you do?

One word: *sustenance.*

When I first started dieting in high school at age fifteen, I thought that diets were something you do for about a week or two, and then you arrive at the maintenance phase, which meant (or so I thought) that the weight stayed off. Now I know that maintenance is not a destination but a dynamic process. I also know, from both my work and my personal experience, that maintenance is the glue. It holds together your ability to stay clean and lean, cell to soul. And it can be the hardest and most critical phase, as we know from the grim statistics of how most diets fail. We also know how yo-yo dieting is actually worse for you than never dieting at all, because it wrecks

your metabolism. But maintenance—or as I prefer to call it, sustenance—can also be the most exciting phase, because you are creating new habits that will make you live a longer, leaner, healthier,
and happier life.

You probably won't be surprised to learn that I offer a new way of
approaching the sustenance phase. Instead of looking at this phase
as a time to rest on your laurels and resume the eating habits that
led you to this book in the first place, I want to harness the power
of your newly clean body and mind, and direct that power toward
taking your health to a whole new level.

I like to think of the twenty-one days of your Hormone Reset
as your debutante ball. You've worked hard to prepare for that
moment—the dress, the hair, the venue, the flowers, the dance
moves. But once the party is over, the real work of becoming an
adult begins. In the same way, once your Hormone Reset is over, the
real work of sustaining your newfound clean body and weight loss
begins. Just as a teenager has a mentor to lead her on her journey,
you have me to guide you on this new path.

## The Science Behind Sustenance

Of course, I have a scientific basis for my rules of sustenance. In a
nutshell, keeping your insulin balanced is the gateway to sustaining
your weight for life. You may not have lost all the weight you want
to release, but I recommend that you perform your Hormone Reset
each quarter (i.e., every three months). Remember the scales that
represent divine justice? One of the depictions shows the goddess
Themis with a sword and a scale. Think of insulin—in balance—as
your powerful sword.

Your problem is hormonal. All paths of fatness lead back to that
rascal hormone, insulin. Yet just as you can reset your insulin in
as little as seventy-two hours, you can ruin it again in just as much

time. So the key to maintenance and preventing weight regain is to keep insulin in its sweet spot: not too high and not too low.

The idea that weight gain is hormonal is a mind bender for most people, so I want to reiterate that you should focus on your seven hormones of metabolism instead of the faulty notion of paying attention only to calories in and calories out. Put another way, positive energy balance (more calories into the body than out) describes what happens when someone gets fat but not *why* he or she gets fat. The "why" is hormones, as we discovered together.

DR. SARA'S SECRET TO AVOID WEIGHT REGAIN

*When it comes to maintaining weight loss, "big doors swing on little hinges" (as W. Clement Stone—businessman, philanthropist, and self-help book author—famously said). What are the little hinges that can lead us to success? Regrettably, the studies on weight regain are ambiguous and poorly designed. Among the studies that are available, the data show that roughly 20 percent of people who lose weight are able to maintain it for one year.[1] It's as if the brain is wired to make you regain weight, so the trick is to reverse the increased appetite and the decrease in resting and exercise-induced metabolic rates. Since the problem of weight gain and regain is hormonal, not caloric, I believe we can do better with maintenance when we really zero in on the little hinges that swing big doors.*

## Dr. Sara's Three Rules of Sustenance

1. *Eat enough protein.* If you don't get enough protein in your diet, you get hungry, start eating more refined carbs, and regain weight. Science shows that insufficient protein leads to weight

regain, and the corollary is true as well—that additional protein prevents weight regain.[2] Women with adrenal dysregulation often don't get enough protein. Keep in mind that if you love to snack, eating sufficient protein also keeps you from getting the munchies.

2. *Avoid refined carbs.* Eating foods with a low-glycemic index/load leads to lower fasting insulin and inflammation—and that's a good thing for getting lean.[3] Refined carbohydrates, not calories, make you fat. Avoid the bad or fat-boosting carbs—sugars, starches, bread, pizza, refined flour, and pasta. In general, the fewer carbs you eat, the leaner you'll be. Protein and fat are essential to your health; carbs are not. Reducing calories won't work for fat loss unless you cut back on carbs. If you don't, you will be hungry and your metabolism will slow down. This is a key problem with most restrictive diets and why they fail. We don't want that, so no more restricting calories. As you've learned, refined carbs that are rapidly digested (and low in fiber) are one of the likely food-based causes of inflammation, heart disease, maybe even cancer. All told, they create a bad neighborhood for your DNA.

3. *Keep your eyes on net carbs and triglycerides.* The best evidence does not prove that saturated fat clogs your arteries. The true enemy is triglycerides, the fat your liver makes like crazy when you're overeating carbohydrates and other low-fiber sources of fructose. That's why I recommend you continue to eat foods like nutrient-dense vegetables (one pound per day), clean and anti-inflammatory proteins (such as crustaceans and cold-water fish), and healthy fats (such as coconut oil and ghee from grass-fed cows).

## Your Dashboard

Pilots rely on their navigational controls to monitor speed, elevation, fuel usage, and pressure. You have a dashboard too. When you're willing to change the root causes of your broken metabolism—from estrogen dominance to slow detoxification—you have the controls right under your fingertips, and the evidence documented in your journal.

Your dashboard leverages the fact that your neurotransmitters and hormones work together. You can bring your whole dashboard into a safe zone by recalibrating how you eat, sleep, move, and think. No emergency oxygen mask required.

Here are the instruments and levers that stay on my dashboard, and I work at them every day:

1. *Start your day with a shake.* We know from the National Weight Control Registry that eating breakfast is essential to maintaining weight loss. We also know that food intolerances are on the rise, so I recommend that you continue to start your day right and set yourself up for success by drinking a medicinal shake. Choose a protein powder for the shake that's anti-inflammatory: free of gluten and dairy, and low in sugar (less than 5 grams of sugar per serving). Watch out for whey, too, if you find you're intolerant.

2. *Dial in your macronutrients.* Our knowledge base of what helps keep weight off has changed over time. Now the best information is that successful losers keep it off by limiting refined carbohydrates and eating more healthy proteins and fats.[4] In fact, since 1995, when we first started tracking the people who are successful at maintaining weight loss, the number of people on a low-carb diet (defined as less than 90 grams per day) has nearly tripled, from 6 to 17 percent. Successful losers are eating more fat—up from 24 to 29 percent of total calories—and

saturated fat consumption has increased from 12 to 154 grams per day. What does that mean for you?

- *Keep your total net carbs between 20 and 49 grams per day.* When you want to maintain your weight, inch up to between 50 and 99 grams per day. Eat slow carbs, particularly vegetables, sweet potatoes, and plantains. (Read labels to count grams of carbs. Also see Measurement #9 on page 32 for a description of how to calculate net carbs.) In my opinion, lower levels of carbohydrates may be risky if you have thyroid or adrenal issues—which most women have! Eat your pound of vegetables per day, drink your shake, and have an occasional roasted sweet potato! I eat 3 ounces of sweet potato at dinner twice each week and find it helps my sleep and adrenal function.

- *For protein, get about 75 to 125 grams per day.* Remember that two eggs contain 13 grams of protein, and 4 ounces of chicken breast has 25 grams.

- *For healthy fats, aim for approximately 30 to 50 percent of total calories per day.*

3. *Crowd out the junk.* This habit works really well when you have a tendency (or outright hard addiction) to certain foods, like sugar, alcohol, or caffeine. You must continue to eat good quantities of healthy food each day—crowd out the physical junk or bad food. I think of it as the 80/20 rule: aim for 80 percent vegetables and 20 percent clean protein. Remember that protein makes you satisfied, and insufficient protein makes you crave carbohydrates. Our goal is to make sure you get enough of the fun, yummy, and nutrient-dense whole foods so you're not hungry for those frenemies (yummy-looking things that are bad for you). As an example, drink a shake for breakfast, and plan your lunch and dinner to be low in sugar. Eat a large salad with a clean protein (fish, shrimp, or chicken), and continue to eat one pound (or more) of vegetables each day. Additionally,

I want you to crowd out the emotional junk, or what scientists call "internal disinhibition"—the thoughts and feelings that derail you from eating the best fuel possible. Having strategies in place, such as the Cell to Soul Practices in chapters 3 through 10, will help you get and stay lean.[5]

4. *Keep measuring.* This habit ensures continuous metabolic accountability and improvement. I challenge you to find the top five measurements that track your progress best, and keep them in mind as a list that you review daily (steps, sleep) and weekly (waist and hip circumferences, blood sugar, body fat, pH). Here are a few more details about how these measurements help support your maintenance:

   • *pH.* New research suggests when you're too acidic from high stress and eating acidifying foods, you gain weight.[6] This may be particularly true in women.[7]

   • *Blood sugar.* Check this once a week so that you can calibrate your blood sugar before it gets out of hand. Ideally your fasting blood sugar is 70–85 mg/dL.

   • *Waist and hip circumferences.* Science shows that your hip measurement is the best estimate of fat mass.[8] Measure weekly.

   • *Blood panel.* Getting this evaluation once every three to six months gives you important data on your hormone levels, such as thyroid. See Resources for where to get blood panels drawn, but the best option is to order labs through your health professional.

5. *Rotate your food.* If you found in Reentry that you had a mild reaction to a food, you may decide to continue to eat it, but in rotation. (If your reaction was moderate to severe, you should completely remove that food.) Eating the same food day after day makes you more likely to develop an allergy and more serious adverse reactions. But if you only eat a food once every four days, a reaction is far less likely to occur. From the reset

chapters (especially Grain Free and Dairy Free), you know that grains and dairy are the most common allergenic foods. Even if you didn't have a reaction to them during this round of your Hormone Reset, you may in the future. Be vigilant and limit your risk by rotating these foods.

6. *Master your sleep.* Recent evidence shows that sleep is crucial to staying sensitive to insulin. If you skimp on sleep, you are more likely to overeat the next day. When you have less REM (rapid eye movement) sleep, you lose insulin sensitivity.[9] The bottom line: mind your sleep so you don't fall down a hormonal flight of stairs and regain weight. I recommend eight hours per night.

7. *Repeat your Hormone Reset every three to six months.* I tell the women who join my online course of the Hormone Reset that life is a series of "detox, retox, detox," meaning I don't expect you to be perfect when it comes to food. However, what works for me and for the vast majority of women is to make the Hormone Reset as a system reboot once every three to six months, to cultivate body awareness, drop pounds, and get lean and clean. Learn more and consider joining the next online event at www.HormoneReset.com/detox.

When it comes to your habit dashboard, remember the ideas from chapter 2 about how habits ideally will replace your reliance on willpower. I wish willpower were consistent all day long, but the truth is willpower fades over the course of the day, which is a major problem for those of us with food dependency.

## Camp Sustenance

Whether you want to get and stay lean because of vanity or sanity, because your doctor told you that you must, or because you just want to fit into your wedding dress, we have good science from the

National Weight Control Registry that informs the rules of maintenance. The registry shows that over a decade its members lost 10 percent of their body weight—and 87 percent have maintained it for more than ten years.[10] In order to be eligible for the registry, adults must have lost at least 30 pounds and kept it off for a year. On average, a woman in the registry (and 80 percent in the registry are women) is forty-five years in age and weighs 145 pounds.

What I find fascinating is that the registry members fall into one of four camps,[11] and my suspicion is that these camps are hormonally and genetically determined.

1. *Stable Mables.* This group includes more than 50 percent of the members. They are stable in weight and are healthy, exercise aggressively, and are very content with their weight.

2. *Strugglers.* Twenty-seven percent of members fit into the second camp. They've struggled with weight since childhood and rely on the greatest number of strategies and resources to stay in their target weight zone. Not surprisingly, many people in this camp describe feeling high stress and depression.

3. *Pink Clouders.* This represents 13 percent of the members, and they were successful at weight loss the first time they tried. Out of the four camps, they are the least likely to have been overweight as kids, have the longest duration of weight maintenance, and have the least difficulty controlling their weight. (I don't know many of these people!)

4. *Restrictors.* Slightly less than 10 percent of the members, restrictors are the least likely to use exercise to control their weight, are older, eat fewer meals, and report more health problems. In other words, they restrict their food instead of exercising.

Take a moment to reflect on which camp you fit into. Once you do, you can use that information to guide your maintenance strategies.

When I learned about the four camps of people who maintain their weight loss for years, I got curious about the specific strategies registry members use to sustain weight loss. That is, what are the little hinges that successfully swing big weight loss maintenance doors for people? The most effective strategies are:[12]

- **maintaining high levels of consistent exercise** (about one hour per day in 90 percent of registry members—in fact, this is more important to prevent weight *regain* than to prevent weight *gain*;[13] another study showed that bursts of ten minutes of moderate-to-vigorous exercise are linked to greater maintenance of weight loss[14]);

- **eating breakfast** regularly;

- **self-monitoring** (75 percent of registry members weigh themselves at least once per week);

- **minimizing TV** (62 percent of registry members watch less than ten hours of TV each week); and

- **maintaining a consistent eating pattern** across weekdays, weekends, and holidays.

I agree with all of those techniques. Interestingly, eating more fat and experiencing disinhibition around food were linked to greater weight regain, but the amount of physical activity was not.[15] That tells me you must pay attention to fat (not too much, not too little), you should avoid your trigger foods, and you don't need to exercise fiendishly for maintenance to work. In my opinion, a healthy breakfast, burst exercise, self-monitoring, and consistency keep these folks lean—and these habits can keep you lean too!

## Creating a Low-Stress Lifestyle

Recently, I went on a trip to Point Reyes, California, which is a nature lover's dream destination. It offers great hiking, kayaking, cycling, horseback riding, and swimming, and it's one of the best places in the country to bird-watch. The light at the end of the day is luminous year-round, and the landscape makes my heart sing and my adrenals smile. It's low stress, and it's good for my body.

After I visit a place like this, I wonder how I can take that sense of peace and bring it back home to my "real" life, filled with a husband, children, a mortgage, and a household to run. I know that a life filled with nothing but bird-watching and hiking is unrealistic. But my goal is to bring back some of the calm I feel in Point Reyes so it's not all or nothing: total stress until I escape and crash for a few days in nature.

Behavioral economist Dan Ariely, PhD, said, "If we understood our cognitive limitations in the same way that we understand our physical limitations . . . we could design a better world." His statement applies to your Hormone Reset; it's a mind-over-mouth game.

Creating a low-stress lifestyle takes some planning. I've found that it's easy to get swept away in the day-to-day world, and a big part of me loves the excitement and energy that permeates my work and my life. I've found a few helpful things to create this kind of lower-stress life, and I want to share them with you. You might want to start incorporating one or more of these into your routine and see where you land.

**Meditate.** I've said it before and I'll say it again. If you can't quit your job or run away to Hawaii, meditation is one of the best things you can do to create inner calm. Clearing your mind of the clutter is as important as taking out the garbage so the kitchen doesn't start to smell. It doesn't take much. Get up ten minutes earlier than you usually do and sit on a cushion. (I have a meditation app that makes a lovely Tibetan bell sound to signify the beginning and end of my meditation.) Take a few deep breaths before settling in. Then begin. Simply watch your thoughts as they arise, and then let them go with your out breath.

**Make cutbacks.** When I look at my life, it's hard to see places to cut back. I don't want to skimp on time with my kids or husband, with my girlfriends, or in my work. I love all of these things. But I've found that I have to look at the nature of these activities and discover ways to modify them to meet my needs for low stress. For example, instead of taking my kids on an all-day outing, I might choose to stay home with them in our pajamas and dance or play a board game. With my work, I might choose to delegate more work to others or cut back one afternoon. I say "probably not" to more queries for my time, so that I have more time to remind myself not to "overcare"—a term popularized by Doc Childre, founder of the Institute of HeartMath—when the mind and emotions cross the line of balanced care and get too attached to and bogged down with whomever or whatever you're caring about.[16]

**Assess the drive.** Commuting and chauffeuring can take a toll. Examine your driving time, and see if there are ways to cut back: carpool, take public transportation, look for a new job, telecommute one day a week. I believe that driving is a major contributor to stress, not to mention that it can take a toll on your body, the planet, and your valuable time.

**Banish the vampires.** Emotional vampires suck the energy right out of you. I want you to think about the vampires in your life, people who make you feel depleted, insecure, or just plain angry. You don't need to hang onto these people. You can wean them from your life, just as you do with sugar.

**Plug into passion.** I don't want to add more to your plate, but in certain cases low stress means adding something you love to your life. Creativity is a life energy that pulses through us; when we don't have it, we can feel low energy and stressed. Figure out what activities you can turn to when you feel stressed: knitting, hiking, painting, poetry writing? Many women let their passions slip away to overcare for others. I'm asking you to reclaim your passion. It will not only benefit you but also benefit everyone around you.

**Schedule in relaxation.** I have a firm rule: I must set aside thirty minutes a day for relaxation or stress relief. Sometimes I run, often I listen to guided meditation on my iPhone, or go for an ambling walk. If I'm ambitious, I'll join a friend for a barre fitness class. It doesn't matter what it is, just that you do it. No excuses: you would easily spend thirty minutes on a phone call or at the coffee shop, so I know you can find the time. Think of this like a reservoir: each time it rains, the reservoir fills up. No rain means no water. If the reservoir is empty, there will be nothing when you are the thirstiest. In the same way, when you practice relaxation, you will be filling up your inner reservoir so that in times of intense stress, you will know how to access a relaxed state of mind.

**Connect to spirit.** One of the key ways to create a low-stress lifestyle is to realize the critical role that your spiritual journey plays in healing your metabolism. When there's no time for your spiritual life, it's more likely that you'll become dependent again on food as a way to fill the void, and you'll regain weight. Figure out what kind of spiritual practice works for you to keep from letting that happen. It could be something I've listed previously, such as meditation or walking in nature. Or it could be praying, joining a spiritual community, or reading inspirational texts. Whatever it is, pick something and make a commitment to conscious contact with a Higher Power of your understanding.

## Supplements

As you sustain your progress with your Hormone Reset, I have a supplement to recommend. While I hope you now understand that baking your child a cake is not as loving as you might think, occasionally we want a treat. For those situations, try a carb blocker that contains *Phaseolus vulgaris*, an extract from white kidney beans. Take it thirty minutes before eating foods that are higher in carbohydrates, such as pumpkin, sweet potatoes, yams, or if you must, the occasional chocolate cake.

## Cell to Soul Practice

When I was in a program for food addiction, I heard a great parable. I tried to find its origin, and my research suggests it may have originated with Native Americans, but it was also described by the Reverend Billy Graham.[17] I want to share it with you because it helped me with maintenance, and I know it will help you too.

My sponsor told me that inside all of us exists a power struggle between a white dog and a black dog. The white dog represents peace, joy, love, acceptance, truth, compassion, and faith. The black dog represents anger, resentment, hate, fear, insecurity, doubt, superiority, and ego. Typically, the black dog will dominate if you're unaware. Which dog will win the internal fight for control of your body and mind? The one that you feed!

The white dog is fed in many ways, such as:

- planning your meals one day in advance so that you're not relying on willpower and a last-minute scramble to feed yourself;
- nurturing yourself and claiming at least a minimal, effective self-care regimen;
- getting regular exercise;
- cultivating body awareness—hitting the pause button with meditation, yoga, and the Cell to Soul Practices featured in this book;
- having meaningful conversations with people you love;

- talking with like-minded friends about your vulnerabilities, and tapping into the collective wisdom about how to address them; and
- intentionally choosing a low-stress life, instead of letting yourself get taken over by stress that is actually under your control.

In other words, the white dog is your Higher Self. When you take your white dog off the leash, she is calm and friendly. She doesn't bite your neighbor or otherwise behave out of control. Amazingly, when you feed your white dog, your black dog calms down, too.

On the other hand, your black dog gets fed in opposite ways, by:

- having a stressful day;
- cutting corners on your sleep;
- waiting too long to eat;
- overeating;
- eating foods that don't serve you;
- leaving food choices to the last minute;
- eating foods that are triggers, such as sugar, grains, and dairy;
- pretending you've got it all figured out and don't need any help; and
- not pursuing your unique abilities and passions.

When you let your black dog off the leash, she goes nuts—barking, biting, pooping and peeing all over the place, and generally destroying your home and upsetting the neighbors.

The bottom line: feed your white dog. It will power your maintenance and provide the momentum you need to keep the weight off and find lasting success.

## Notes from Hormone Resetters

When I take a group of women through the Hormone Reset Diet, I love to hear all the different ways women feel back home in their body once they are finished with the seven resets. There are many variations on how this feels to a woman, and I offer the following descriptions so that you can see which resonates most with you, now that you're at the end of your Hormone Reset.

"I love to reside in this sacred temple." —*Arti*

"When your body and mind are in sync, you feel like you're unstoppable, vibrant, and energetic, but in a calm and grounded way. It's nirvana!"—*Michele*

"When I'm at home in my body, I feel fully awake and appreciative of all life has to offer and the desire to receive it."—*Sherry*

I can relate to each of these women, and I imagine the same may be true for you. They point to what's lost for us as women when we get too busy to listen to our bodies and use our inner guidance. When we take the time to clean the slate, we feel amazing. "It feels like a warm, sunny day," said one woman after the Hormone Reset. "I feel a deep sense of calm, contentment, and happiness—physically and emotionally." It's up to you to make that choice: Do you want it to be stormy and rainy, or do you want a wonderful sunshine to warm your body? Each day, you have the chance to control your inner weather. I encourage you to choose the warm sunshine instead of mud and thunderclouds. That way you can deal more gracefully with the inevitable winds of change that will come.

## Final Word

Over the course of your Hormone Reset, you've learned firsthand about the foods that tend to cause harm through allergies, intolerances, hormone imbalance, broken metabolism, and fat-loss resistance. After elimination and provocation, you are empowered to listen even more closely to your body and make the best decisions about which foods serve you.

I hope you know by now that this is about so much more than weight loss. It's about mastery over your life. When you feel energetic, strong, and in touch with your body, wonderful things can happen. Now that you are no longer bloated and cranky, obsessed and neurotic, or guilty and self-loathing about your body, you can finally focus on your deepest hopes and dreams, your purpose in life, your voice, your place in the world. You can discover what makes you feel most alive and awake. It's huge.

Like the thousands of women who've gone through the Hormone Reset, I hope you feel enchanted by your body and continue to cultivate the awareness that you need to maintain your progress with grace. Please count on me as a resource for you at any point at www .HormoneReset.com. Even if you live far away, imagine that I'm there, by your side, as you go food shopping or exercise. When you come to a crossroads, and you most certainly will, ask yourself what I might do or say. I hope this provides you with some guidance and insight. Thank you for your commitment, sharing this time with me, and taking vital steps to create and sustain your progress.

I will leave you with an image of the lotus flower. You might have noticed one floating on a pond or seen a picture. This exquisite and fragrant flower is amazing: it literally grows up from the mud, spreading its petals toward the sun, full of inner intelligence and subtle energy from the inside out.

You are the lotus flower. No matter where you've come from or what you've been through, you have the potential to break through toward the light, to cultivate awareness, to accept where you are and where you are headed—and to bloom. You are gentle yet strong, determined, and beautiful. I honor your bravery and commitment. Once you've seen the light, I hope you decide to dwell and thrive in it for many years to come.

# Recipes

Food should be delicious and nourishing, and it should keep you feeling energized from your cells to your soul. These recipes are designed to heal your metabolism and to be easy for busy people to prepare.

## Dr. Sara's Basic Vanilla Shake

*Geek Out with Dr. Sara:* Protein shakes are a great opportunity to consume effortlessly a serving of nutrient-rich, fresh vegetables. (Lightly steam them if you have thyroid issues to reduce the goitrogenic or thyroid-slowing effect.) I always add at least a cup of greens, usually frozen kale, to my shakes. Some people dislike kale because it is fibrous and bitter, but I find that the flavor is easily masked in this drink.

*Makes 1 serving*

2 scoops *Dr. Sara's Vanilla Shake* (or similar protein powder)
2 scoops *Dr. Sara's Fiber* (or similar)
1 tablespoon cashew or almond butter

1 cup unsweetened coconut milk, unsweetened almond milk, or
filtered water (add more liquid if you like your shake thinner)
4 or 5 ice cubes

Blend all ingredients in a blender until smooth.

## Dr. Sara's Basic Chocolate Shake

*Makes 1 serving*

2 scoops *Dr. Sara's Chocolate Shake* (or similar protein powder)
2 scoops *Dr. Sara's Fiber* (or similar)
1 cup unsweetened coconut , unsweetened almond milk, or filtered
water
4 or 5 ice cubes
½ tablespoon maca powder to support estrogen metabolism
(optional)*
1 tablespoon cacao nibs to sprinkle on top for a little crunch
(optional)
1 tablespoon medium-chain triglyceride (MCT) oil to boost fat
burning (optional)

Blend all ingredients in a blender until smooth.

*See *The Hormone Cure*, page 191, for more information, or go to www.thehormonecure
book.com.

## Detox Shake

*Geek Out with Dr. Sara:* Unsweetened almond milk has 50 percent
more calcium than dairy milk! Getting off dairy never tasted so good.

*Makes 1 serving*

2 scoops *Dr. Sara's Vanilla Shake* (or similar protein powder)
2 scoops *Dr. Sara's Fiber* (or similar)
1 cup almond milk or filtered water (add more liquid if you like
your shake thinner)

1 cup kale
1 tablespoon MCT oil
4 or 5 ice cubes

Blend all ingredients in a high-powered blender (for instance, Vita-mix, Blendtec, Magic Bullet, or NutriBullet—see Resources) until smooth.

## Mint Chocolate Chip Shake

*Geek Out with Dr. Sara:* Here's a detoxifying drink that is as healthy as a tonic and as nutritious as a balanced meal, and it tastes like dessert! Cacao nibs are roasted cacao beans, the essence of chocolate.

*Makes 1 serving*

2 scoops *Dr. Sara's Chocolate Shake* (or similar protein powder)
1½ cups unsweetened coconut milk (or less to make your shake thicker)
1 cup fresh chopped mint leaves
½ cup fresh dandelion greens
¼ cup raw cacao nibs
4 or 5 ice cubes
1 tablespoon cacao nibs (optional)
1 fresh mint leaf (optional)

Blend all ingredients in a high-powered blender until smooth. Garnish with cacao nibs and a mint leaf.

## Sunflower Chia Shake

*Geek Out with Dr. Sara:* Sunflower seeds are rich in vitamin B6, which helps you make more of the happy brain chemical, serotonin, and reduces your risk of premenstrual syndrome.

*Makes 1 serving*

- 2 scoops *Dr. Sara's Vanilla Shake* (or similar protein powder)
- 2 tablespoons chia seeds, soaked in water overnight
- 2 tablespoons unsweetened sunflower seeds (or sunflower butter)
- 1 cup unsweetened coconut milk, unsweetened almond milk, or filtered water
- 1 cup kale leaves
- 4 or 5 ice cubes
- 2 teaspoons freshly minced ginger root (optional)

Blend all ingredients in a high-powered blender until smooth. Enjoy!

## Hazelnut Chocolate Spice Shake

*Makes 1 serving*

- 2 scoops *Dr. Sara's Chocolate Shake* (or similar protein powder)
- 1-inch piece of fresh ginger, peeled and chopped
- 1 tablespoon pure cacao powder
- 1 tablespoon raw cacao nibs
- 1 tablespoon cashew butter
- 1 cup raw kale*
- 1 tablespoon turmeric
- 1 cup unsweetened hazelnut milk
- 2 tablespoons chia seeds, soaked (optional)

Blend all ingredients in a high-powered blender until smooth.

*I buy kale, wash and chop it, and freeze it for shakes.

**THE HORMONE RESET BEVERAGES**

## Tulsi Tea

*Geek Out with Dr. Sara:* Tulsi, or holy basil, is an herb used in Ayurvedic medicine for its healing and stimulating effects. Replace your morning cup of coffee with this invigorating tea, and you may also be helping to reduce the damage that years of coffee consumption have inflicted. Tulsi has been shown to be a powerful anti-inflammatory and has properties that may prevent ulcers.

*Makes 2 to 3 servings*

   8 tablespoons dried organic tulsi
   4 tablespoons dried dandelion leaves
   4 cups boiling water
   4 cups cool water

Steep Tulsi and dandelion leaves in boiling water for at least 30 minutes. Once tea has become quite strong, strain leaves and add cool water. Tulsi tea is traditionally served at room temperature.

Adapted with permission from Jessica Theroux's Tulsi Tea.


## Love Your Liver Tonic
.........................................................................................................................

*Geek Out with Dr. Sara:* This tonic is an anti-inflammatory power-house. Turmeric, ginger, cinnamon, chard, and beets are all particularly potent combatants of inflammation. Remember that blended veggies count toward your daily pound. Just be sure to drink the pulp by using a high-powered blender (see Resources)!

*Makes 3 to 4 servings*

   6 cups filtered water
   2 medium beets, peeled and sliced
   2 cinnamon sticks
   2-inch piece of fresh ginger, peeled and chopped
   2-inch piece of fresh turmeric, peeled and chopped
   1 cup broccoli sprouts
   4 or 5 large leaves of red chard
   8 to 10 leaves of dandelion greens

½ cup fresh mint leaves
Juice of one red grapefruit

1. Place water, beets, and cinnamon sticks in a large pot over high heat.
2. Bring to a boil, and cook until the beets are tender, approximately 20 to 30 minutes.
3. Strain the beets, and discard the water and cinnamon sticks.
4. Blend the beets, ginger, turmeric, broccoli sprouts, chard, dandelion greens, mint, and grapefruit juice in a high-powered blender; add the mixture to the pot.
5. Let the tonic heat over a low flame for another hour or two.
6. Serve warm or cold.


## Quick Green Tonic

If you find yourself having trouble consuming a pound of vegetables a day, try blending them into a tonic. This potent dose of antioxidants goes down quicker than a salad and travels better. I use my blender for tonics, juices, and smoothies because blending whole vegetables doesn't remove the fiber as juicing does. Not to mention, blending is faster, easier, and less messy!

*Makes 1 serving*

½ medium Shepherd or Hass avocado
½ cup watercress leaves
1-inch piece of fresh ginger, peeled and chopped
1-inch piece of fresh turmeric root, peeled and chopped
½ cup radish sprouts
Juice of two limes
1 cup filtered water
3 or 4 ice cubes
1 tablespoon of MCT oil (optional)

Blend all ingredients in a high-powered blender until smooth. Energizing!

## Tea and Collagen Frappe

. . . . . . . . . . . . . . . . . . . . . . . . . . . . . . . . . . . . . . . . . . . . . . . . . . . . . . . . . . . . . . . . . . . . . . . . . . . . . . . . . . . . . . . . .

*Makes 1 serving*

- Brewed tea
- 3 tablespoons collagen (clean protein; see Resources)
- 1 tablespoon MCT oil

Blend all ingredients in a blender for 30 seconds.

### THE HORMONE RESET SALADS

## Delicata Squash Salad

. . . . . . . . . . . . . . . . . . . . . . . . . . . . . . . . . . . . . . . . . . . . . . . . . . . . . . . . . . . . . . . . . . . . . . . . . . . . . . . . . . . . . . . . .

*Geek Out with Dr. Sara:* Don't toss the seeds from your delectable delicata squash! Winter squash seeds provide omega-6 fatty acids. To preserve these vital oils, roast your seeds at a low temperature for a short time—about 160°F for 15 minutes. Toss with cinnamon or cayenne for a crunchy salad topping or afternoon snack.

*Makes 6 servings*

- 4 or 5 delicata squash
- 2 teaspoons melted coconut oil, divided
- 2 teaspoons sea salt, divided
- 4 shallots
- ¾ cup sunflower seeds
- ⅓ cup olive oil
- 3 tablespoons lemon juice
- ½ teaspoon salt

1 teaspoon organic, hardwood-derived xylitol (make sure it's not
   made from GMO corn)
2 tablespoons warm water
½ cup chopped cilantro

1. Preheat the oven to 375°F.
2. Slice the delicata squash into thin slices or cubes. Toss them in a
   large bowl with half of the coconut oil and salt. Spread the squash
   in a single layer on a baking sheet.
3. Dice the shallots, and toss them with the remaining coconut oil
   and salt. Spread the shallots on a separate baking sheet.
4. Bake the squash and the shallots for 30 to 45 minutes.
5. Meanwhile, blend the sunflower seeds, olive oil, lemon juice,
   salt, xylitol, and warm water in a food processor or blender until
   smooth. You may want to add more or less xylitol or salt, depending on taste.
6. Toss the squash, shallots, and cilantro in a large bowl, and serve
   with the dressing on top.

## Arugula Salad with Wild Mushrooms and Dairy-Free Brie

*Geek Out with Dr. Sara:* Tree nuts and nut milks make an excellent
base for dairy-free cheese. Whereas soy-based fake cheeses are often
rubbery and bland, nuts provide the rich texture and complex flavor
we expect to find in dairy cheese. Rich in healthy fats and vitamins,
nuts are also more nutritious than soybeans. This recipe calls for an
artisanal variety of nut cheese, which is relatively simple to make
at home and a far cry from the processed soy product we typically
associate with dairy-free cheese.

*Makes 4 to 6 servings*

3 tablespoons rendered duck fat
1 small clove of garlic, minced

1 cup wild mushroom medley, chopped
2 tablespoons red wine vinegar
1 tablespoon olive oil
½ teaspoon truffle salt
½ teaspoon black pepper
3 cups baby arugula
6 ounces Creamy Dairy-Free Brie (page 282), or other soft dairy-free
   cheese such as Kite Hill White Alder (available at Whole Foods)
¼ cup radish sprouts

1. Heat the duck fat over medium heat in a small skillet, sauté the garlic and mushrooms until soft.
2. Transfer the mushrooms, garlic, and remaining fat from the pan to a small bowl. Whisk in the red wine vinegar, olive oil, truffle salt, and black pepper to create the dressing.
3. Drizzle the dressing over the arugula in a large bowl, and toss until coated.
4. Serve the salad with thin slices of cheese on top, and garnish with radish sprouts.

## Watercress and Arugula Salad with Green Goddess Dressing

*Geek Out with Dr. Sara:* This salad contains ingredients rich in beneficial phytonutrients, specifically sulforaphane, which aids in cleansing the body of toxins because it activates enzymes in the liver essential to detoxification.

*Makes 4 to 6 servings*

1 shallot
1 garlic clove
3 tablespoons white wine vinegar
2 whole anchovies
½ avocado
⅓ cup full-fat coconut milk

½ cup olive oil
¼ cup finely chopped parsley
3 tablespoons finely chopped basil
1 tablespoon dried tarragon
1 tablespoon dried oregano
Salt and pepper to taste
3 cups baby arugula
1 cup watercress leaves
4 or 5 watermelon radishes, sliced thin
½ cup sprouts

1. Blend the shallot, garlic, white wine vinegar, anchovies, and avocado in a blender or food processor until smooth.
2. With the blender on low, slowly drizzle the coconut milk and olive oil into the mixture.
3. Transfer the dressing to a small bowl, and whisk them together with the parsley, basil, tarragon, and oregano. Add salt and pepper to taste.
4. Toss the dressing with the arugula, watercress, radishes, and sprouts in a large bowl.

Adapted from Alice Waters's Green Goddess Dressing. Alice Waters, *In the Green Kitchen* (New York: Clarkston Potter, 2010), p. 14.

## Quinoa, Avocado, and Chickpea Salad

*Geek Out with Dr. Sara:* Quinoa is probably the world's healthiest seed (not a grain). Unlike cereal grains, quinoa contains healthy fats, protein, and many valuable phytonutrients.

*Makes 4 servings*

2 cups cooked quinoa
1 15-ounce can chickpeas (garbanzo beans—look for a BPA-free can!)
1 large avocado, sliced
1 cucumber, chopped

1 cup cherry tomatoes, halved (unless you are restricting
   nightshades)
Juice of 1 lemon
2 tablespoons extra-virgin olive oil
Salt and pepper to taste

Toss all ingredients together in a large bowl, and serve. This salad will keep in the refrigerator for three days if you omit the avocado until ready to serve.

## Kale and Beet Salad with Red Wine Vinaigrette

*Geek Out with Dr. Sara:* The red pigment found in vegetables such as beets, chard stems, and rhubarb comes from phytonutrients known as betalains. If you have ever peeled a beet with your bare hands, you know what a potent amount of this pigment the root vegetable contains. Betalains promote detoxification in the body by enabling the production of enzymes in the liver.

*Makes 4 to 6 servings*

*Dressing:*
   3 tablespoons red wine vinegar
   2 tablespoons olive oil
   1 teaspoon thyme
   ½ teaspoon fennel seeds
   Salt and pepper to taste
*Salad:*
   1 medium beet
   4 or 5 large leaves of dinosaur kale
   Half a head of butter lettuce, chopped
   Quarter of a red onion, thinly sliced

**For dressing:**
Whisk the vinegar, olive oil, thyme, fennel seeds, and salt and pepper together in a small bowl. Set aside.

**For salad:**
1. Cover the beet with water in a medium pan, and bring to a boil.
2. Reduce the heat and simmer until the beet is tender, approximately 20 to 30 minutes.
3. Remove the beet from the pan, and rinse in cold water. Slice off the skin, and cut the flesh into small thin pieces. Set aside.
4. Massage the kale between your fingers until the leaves become bright green and silky in texture. Slice the massaged leaves into thin pieces.
5. Toss the kale, beet, lettuce, and onion together in a large bowl.
6. Top with the dressing, and enjoy!

## Butternut Squash Salad "Squoutons"

When you want a little bit of crispy, carby goodness on top of your salad, try these "croutons" warm over shredded kale and lettuce with sliced red onion and a red wine vinaigrette.

*Makes 4 to 6 servings*

> 1 butternut squash
> 1 tablespoon coconut oil
> 1 teaspoon salt
> ½ teaspoon ground black pepper
> 1 teaspoon cayenne pepper (optional)

1. Preheat the oven to 475°F.
2. Peel the butternut squash, and remove the seeds. Dice into ½-inch square pieces. Toss in a large bowl with oil and spices until each piece is well coated.
3. Line a large baking sheet with aluminum foil, and arrange the squash in a single layer with plenty of room between each small piece.
4. Bake for 20 to 30 minutes. Flip the croutons over using a spatula,

and bake for an additional 5 to 7 minutes or until golden brown and tender on the inside. Enjoy over your favorite salad.

## Thai Coconut Chicken Soup (Tom Kha Gai)

Kaffir lime leaves are sometimes hard to find. The zest and juice of one lime can be substituted.

*Makes 6 to 8 servings*

   2 stalks lemongrass
   1 large piece of Chinese ginger, peeled and chopped
   10 to 12 Kaffir lime leaves
   2 cloves garlic
   2 whole cardamom pods
   6 cups low-sodium chicken broth
   1 pound free-range, organic, boneless chicken breast or thighs, cut
      into 1-inch pieces
   1 cup chopped shiitake mushrooms
   1 13.5-ounce can organic unsweetened coconut milk
   3 tablespoons fish sauce
   Chili oil and cilantro leaves for garnish

1. Remove the base of the lemongrass stalks with a sharp knife, and discard the tough outer layer. Chop the lemongrass stalks into 2-inch pieces, and toss them into a blender with the chopped ginger, Kaffir lime leaves, and garlic cloves.
2. Pulse the blender a few times until most of the ingredients form a pulp.
3. Add the blended ingredients and the cardamom pods to a large stock pan, and cook over medium-high heat for 1 to 2 minutes until fragrant.

4. Add the chicken broth, and bring to a boil. Reduce heat to low, and simmer for 20 to 30 minutes to allow the flavors to infuse.
5. Strain broth through a fine sieve into a large clean pan. Add the chicken and mushrooms to the broth, and simmer for 20 to 25 minutes until the chicken is cooked through.
6. Remove from the heat. Stir in the coconut milk and fish sauce.
7. Garnish with the chili oil and fresh cilantro leaves before serving.

## Creamy Goddess Greens Soup

*Geek Out with Dr. Sara:* The dairy industry would have us believe that milk is an indispensable source of calcium in our diet as calcium is necessary for healthy bones. What the milk advertisements don't tell us is that there are many other sources of calcium besides dairy products, and that the mineral is only one of the building blocks essential for bone health. Vitamins K and D are also crucial ingredients for bone metabolism. Unlike dairy, the vegetables in this soup provide calcium and the vitamins needed to balance and facilitate the body's ability to use calcium—and it tastes as rich and creamy as a dairy-based soup.

*Makes 6 to 8 servings*

2 tablespoons coconut oil
3 cups cauliflower florets, chopped
6 asparagus spears, chopped
2 large shallots
2 cloves garlic
1 cup arugula
1 cup broccoli rabe florets
½ cup watercress leaves
3 cups organic vegetable or free-range chicken broth
¾ cup unsweetened coconut milk
3 tablespoons lemon juice
¼ teaspoon cayenne pepper

1 teaspoon dried rosemary
Salt and pepper to taste

1. Heat the coconut oil in the bottom of a large soup pot over medium heat. Add the cauliflower, asparagus, shallots, and garlic, and cook until the cauliflower is tender and the shallots are translucent.
2. Reduce the heat to low. Stir in the arugula, broccoli rabe, and watercress. Keep stirring over low heat until the leaves have brightened.
3. Add the broth. Working in batches, transfer the soup to a blender, and purée until smooth.
4. Return the soup to the pot over low heat. Stir in the coconut milk, lemon juice, cayenne pepper, rosemary, and salt and pepper. Enjoy!

Adapted from Mark Hyman's Green Goddess Broccoli and Arugula Soup. Mark Hyman, *The Blood Sugar Solution 10-Day Detox Diet: Activate Your Body's Natural Ability to Burn Fat and Lose Weight Fast* (New York: Little Brown and Company, 2014), pp. 276–77.

## THE HORMONE RESET ENTRÉES

## Dr. Sara's Pumpkin Porridge

I agree with Diane Sanfilippo that a warm bowl of porridge in the morning feels supernurturing. Here is an adaptation of a porridge that I learned from her.

*Makes 1 serving*

1 tablespoon pastured ghee (casein-free)
3 tablespoons ground hemp seeds
1 tablespoon ground Marcona almonds
1 tablespoon tahini

½ cup pumpkin purée
½ teaspoon cinnamon
2 tablespoons shredded coconut
1 to 4 tablespoons unsweetened coconut milk
Stevia or xylitol to taste

Heat the ghee in a small pan over low heat. Add the remaining ingredients, adjusting the coconut milk to achieve the desired consistency. Serve warm.

Adapted with permission from Diane Sanfilippo's Grain Free Porridge. Diane Sanfilippo, *Practical Paleo* (Las Vegas: Victory Belt, 2012), p. 252.

## Protein Egg Muffins
........................................................................................................

These high-protein, grain-free muffins are great for when you need to grab breakfast on the fly. Try variations with different meats and vegetables, or substitute kale for chard or add roasted bell peppers for a different flavor.

*Makes 12 servings*

1 teaspoon coconut oil
1 garlic clove, minced
1 cup shredded chard
12 large eggs
½ teaspoon salt
½ teaspoon black pepper
½ teaspoon fennel seeds
1 teaspoon cayenne pepper
¼ cup green onions or shallots, finely chopped
½ pound sausage, bacon, or chicken breast, fully cooked and chopped or shredded into small pieces

1. Preheat the oven to 425°F.
2. Heat the coconut oil in a large frying pan with a tight-fitting lid over medium heat. Add the garlic, and cook for a few minutes until the garlic softens.

3. Add the shredded chard to the pan, and cover. Cook for approximately 3 minutes, until the chard brightens and becomes tender. Strain the chard and rinse with cold water. Set aside.

4. Beat the eggs in a large bowl with the salt, pepper, fennel seeds, and cayenne. Stir in the chard and onions.

5. Line a muffin tin with 12 paper baking cups. Fill each cup halfway with the egg mixture. Spoon a few tablespoons of the chopped meat into each cup. Pour a little more egg on top of each cup to seal the muffin.

6. Bake the muffins for approximately 35 minutes or until the egg sets and becomes golden brown on top.

Adapted with permission from Diane Sanfilippo's Buffalo Chicken Egg Muffins. Diane Sanfilippo, *Practical Paleo* (Las Vegas: Victory Belt, 2012), p. 100.

## Zucchini Noodles with Arugula Pesto

This is one of those miraculous dishes that is both delicious and incredibly healthy. You can choose to skip sautéing the zucchini for a completely raw, vegan, Paleo, and Hormone Reset Diet–friendly meal that is flavorful and filling.

*Makes 4 to 6 servings*

2 large zucchini, or 4 or 5 small zucchini
2 tablespoons full-fat, unsweetened coconut milk
Juice of one lemon
1 teaspoon garlic salt
½ teaspoon black pepper
4 cups fresh arugula
3 tablespoons nutritional yeast
1 or 2 cloves fresh garlic, depending on taste
Zest of one lemon
⅓ cup olive oil
1 tablespoon coconut oil

1. Using a julienne peeler, peel the zucchini lengthwise into long slices. They should look like spaghetti noodles. Set aside.
2. Blend the coconut milk, lemon juice, garlic salt, and pepper in a food processor until smooth. Add the arugula, nutritional yeast, garlic cloves, lemon zest, and olive oil, and blend again until creamy.
3. Heat the coconut oil in a very large skillet over medium-high heat. Add the zucchini noodles. You may need to work in batches, depending on the size of your skillet. Sauté the zucchini until the noodles have just brightened, approximately 4 to 6 minutes.
4. Remove the zucchini from the pan, and serve with pesto.

## Hazelnut-Coconut-Crusted Halibut Fish Sticks

This gluten-free hazelnut and coconut crust is crispier and more flavorful than panko breadcrumbs. Even picky kids love this gourmet version of the classic frozen fish stick.

*Makes 4 servings*

1 cup hazelnut meal (also called hazelnut flour)
½ cup unsweetened coconut flakes
½ teaspoon salt
½ teaspoon black pepper
1½ pounds fresh halibut fillet
1 large egg
2 tablespoons coconut oil

1. Combine the hazelnut meal, coconut, salt, and pepper in a large bowl. Stir well.
2. Rinse the halibut, and pat it dry with a paper towel. Cut the fillet into 1-inch-wide strips.
3. Beat the egg in a separate small bowl.
4. Submerge each piece of fish in the egg, then dip it into the crust mixture and coat well.

5. Heat the coconut oil over medium heat in a large skillet.
6. Fry the fish in the oil for about 2 minutes on each side, or until opaque in the center. Enjoy!

Adapted from Lena Cederham Birnbaum et al. "Halibut Fish Sticks with Dill-Caper Tartar Sauce," *Bon Appetit*, June 2010, 44.

## Dr. Sara's Hormone Reset Crab Cakes

*Geek Out with Dr. Sara:* Crabmeat is rich in nutrients, including the amazing omega-3s, which are great for your brain, heart, and metabolic function. Crab is also a low-risk seafood for mercury content, since it is small in size and low on the food chain. Make sure your crab is very fresh and has no fishy odor. Alternatively, you can use canned wild pink salmon in lieu of fresh crab if crab is not in season.

*Makes 4 to 6 servings*

  4 radishes
  1 small shallot
  1 clove fresh garlic
  2 eggs
  ½ pound fresh crabmeat, fully cooked
  ½ teaspoon rosemary salt
  1 teaspoon dried parsley
  ½ teaspoon paprika
  ½ teaspoon garlic powder
  ½ teaspoon black pepper
  3 to 4 tablespoons ghee or coconut oil

1. Pulse the radishes, shallot, and garlic in a food processor until finely minced.
2. Beat the eggs in a large mixing bowl, and add the minced radishes, shallot, and garlic. Mix in the crabmeat and all the spices.
3. Heat the ghee or oil over medium heat in a large frying pan.

4. Form the crab mixture into small flat cakes, and fry each cake for approximately 5 to 7 minutes on each side, or until well browned and cooked through.
5. Serve on a bed of fresh greens, and enjoy!

Adapted with permission from Diane Sanfilippo's Quick and Easy Salmon Cakes. Diane Sanfilippo, *Practical Paleo* (Las Vegas: Victory Belt, 2012), p. 310.

## Crispy Sweet Potato Wedges

*Geek Out with Dr. Sara:* Sweet potatoes are an excellent source of beta-carotene. Beta-carotene is a fat-soluble vitamin, and studies show that at least 3 to 5 grams of fat are required for delivery to the bloodstream and for the body to convert beta-carotene to vitamin A. In this recipe, the coconut oil provides the fat your body needs to make the most of this vital nutrient in the potato.

*Makes 1 to 2 servings*

1 large organic orange-fleshed sweet potato
1½ tablespoons organic cold-pressed coconut oil
½ teaspoon dried rosemary
Pink Himalayan salt and black pepper to taste
½ teaspoon chili flakes (optional)

1. Preheat the oven to 425°F.
2. Wash the sweet potato, but do not peel it. Cut it into thin wedge-shaped pieces. The thin wedge shape is important for crispiness. Each wedge should have an edge with skin about ½ inch wide.
3. Place the wedges in a large bowl with the coconut oil, rosemary, salt and pepper, and, if desired, chili flakes. Toss to coat all wedges in oil and spices.
4. Spread the wedges evenly in a single layer on a baking sheet. Bake for 15 minutes, then flip each wedge over. Bake for an additional 8 to 10 minutes.

5. Allow the wedges to cool for 5 minutes. Enjoy with unsweetened organic ketchup, mustard, or homemade aioli.

**Variation:** Toss with a clove of minced garlic before baking.

## Ceviche

........................................................................................................

*Geek Out with Dr. Sara:* This exotic Caribbean recipe is surprisingly simple and easy to prepare at home. The citric acid in lime juice is alkalinizing (a good thing for your body) and cures the shrimp, turning it pink as if it were steamed or boiled. Although the shrimp is not exactly raw, it is still important to use very fresh shrimp for this dish.

*Makes 4 to 6 servings*

> 1 pound of fresh raw shrimp, peeled and deveined, tails removed
> ½ cup finely chopped red onion
> 2 to 3 cups fresh-squeezed lime juice
> 2 medium cucumbers
> 2 avocados
> 3 Roma tomatoes, diced
> ½ cup fresh coconut meat, shredded (optional)
> ½ teaspoon organic hot sauce (optional)
> 1 teaspoon sea salt
> 1 teaspoon freshly ground black pepper

1. Dice the shrimp into bite-size pieces, and place them in a large bowl with the chopped onion.
2. Add enough lime juice to cover all the shrimp. Stir gently to ensure all the shrimp are doused in juice.
3. Cover the bowl, and let the shrimp marinate in lime juice for 20 minutes, or until the flesh has turned pink. Stir and inspect the pieces to make sure no gray color remains.

4. While the shrimp is marinating, peel the cucumbers, cut them in half, and scoop out the seeds with a spoon. Chop the cucumbers and avocados into small pieces.

5. Add the cucumber, tomatoes, avocado, and, if desired, coconut to the bowl, and toss. Add the hot sauce, if desired, and the salt and pepper.

6. Enjoy over gluten-free tortilla chips.

## Maca and Pistachio-Crusted Peruvian Sea Bass

The respected Monterey Bay Aquarium Seafood Watch used to recommend avoiding Chilean sea bass (technically, toothfish) because of illegal fishing, but now it says pirate fishing is all but gone. It recommends looking for the blue eco-label of the Marine Stewardship Council. My recommendation: Peruvian sea bass. It's a smaller fish, so it has a lower mercury content. If you prefer, you can substitute your favorite small (low-mercury) fish in this recipe.

*Geek Out with Dr. Sara:* Maca powder is derived from the maca root, a South American superfood. Packed with vitamins, nutrients, and alkaloids that nourish the endocrine system, maca is used in folk medicine as an effective natural stimulant and aphrodisiac. In a recent study of male athletes, participants who consumed maca showed increased physical performance and sexual drive.

*Makes 4 servings*

> 2 tablespoons ghee
> 2 tablespoons coconut oil
> 2 cloves garlic
> 4 Peruvian sea bass fillets
> ½ cup freshly ground pistachios
> ½ cup maca powder
> Zest of two sweet limes
> 1½ teaspoons sea salt
> ½ teaspoon black pepper

1. Preheat the oven to 375°F.
2. Mix the ghee, coconut oil, and garlic in a food processor until evenly combined.
3. Rub each fish fillet with this mixture until it is thickly and evenly coated.
4. Heat a skillet over high heat. Add the fish to brown for 2 to 3 minutes on each side. Remove the fish from the heat, and set aside.
5. Combine the pistachios, maca powder, lime zest, salt, and pepper together in a large bowl.
6. Dip each fillet in this mixture. Use your hands to ensure the fish is covered on all sides with the crumbs.
7. Bake the fish in a shallow baking dish for 8 to 10 minutes until opaque and slightly flaky. Enjoy!

## Ground Turkey Endive Roll-Ups

Endive leaves are a great low-carb substitute for chips, taco shells, or sandwich buns. They keep their shape better than lettuce leaves and have a yummy crisp texture. Try red endive if you would like a less bitter taste.

*Makes 4 servings*

   2 tablespoons coconut oil
   1 pound ground turkey
   1 teaspoon chili powder
   1 teaspoon garlic powder
   ¼ teaspoon onion powder
   ¼ teaspoon red pepper flakes
   ¼ teaspoon dried oregano
   ¼ teaspoon paprika
   1 teaspoon ground cumin
   1 teaspoon sea salt
   1 teaspoon black pepper
   2 large endives

1. Melt the coconut oil in a large skillet over medium heat. Add the ground turkey and all the spices, and cook until well browned.
2. Separate the endive leaves, and spoon a few tablespoons of ground turkey into each leaf. Serve with dairy-free guacamole or salsa.

Adapted with permission from Diane Sanfilippo's Chinese 5-Spice Turkey Lettuce Cups. Diane Sanfilippo, *Practical Paleo* (Las Vegas: Victory Belt, 2012), p. 272.

## Spaghetti Squash with Kale Pesto

*Geek Out with Dr. Sara:* High in vitamin C and fiber, spaghetti squash is a healthy and tasty alternative to pasta. Vitamin C helps reset progesterone, and the fiber resets your estrogen. My friend Jonathan Bailor, author of the bestseller *The Calorie Myth*, calls spaghetti squash strands "squoodles." One cup of squoodles has approximately 30 grams fewer carbohydrates than gluten-free pasta.

*Makes 10 servings*

  1 organic spaghetti squash
  1 small bunch (approximately 4 cups) of organic kale
  3 tablespoons fresh dill
  ⅓ cup almonds
  Juice of one lemon
  4 tablespoons olive oil
  2 cloves garlic
  1 teaspoon pink Himalayan sea salt
  2 teaspoons freshly ground black pepper

1. Preheat the oven to 375°F.
2. Cut the spaghetti squash in half lengthwise, and scoop out the seeds and pulp. Place one half, cut side down, on a baking sheet. (You can also bake the other side at this time, as cooked squash stores well in the refrigerator.) Bake for 45 minutes.

3. While the squash is baking, blend all the other ingredients together in a food processor or high-powered blender.

4. Once the squash is tender, allow it to cool slightly, then use a fork to separate the fleshy strands from the rind.

5. Stir the strands together with the pesto in a large bowl.

Adapted with permission from Cynthia Pasquella's Kale Walnut Pesto Pasta. Cynthia Pasquella, *The Hungry Hottie Cookbook* (Malibu: Rainy Cat Press, 2012), p. 140.

## Pistachio-Crusted Stuffed Chicken Breasts

This dish is a dressed-up solution to the boring boneless, skinless chicken breast. Dr. Mark Hyman inspired me with the yummy recipes in his book *The Blood Sugar Solution 10-Day Detox Diet*. Be sure to use meat from an organic, free-range bird.

*Makes 4 to 6 servings*

- 4 boneless, skinless chicken breasts
- 2 or 3 leaves of kale
- 4 slices roasted red pepper
- 3 ounces almond cheese
- 2 tablespoons extra-virgin olive oil
- 2 tablespoons cashew butter
- 2 tablespoons lemon juice
- 1 teaspoon sea salt
- ½ teaspoon onion powder
- ½ teaspoon oregano
- ½ teaspoon garlic powder
- ½ teaspoon cumin
- ½ cup pistachios, shells removed
- 4 tablespoons quinoa flakes
- 3 tablespoons coconut oil

1. Preheat the oven to 350°F.
2. Rinse the chicken breasts, and dry them with a paper towel. Slice into the side of each breast at its thickest point to create a pocket for stuffing.
3. Slice the kale leaves and roasted red pepper into thin slices. Shred the almond cheese, and stir together in a small bowl with the kale and peppers. Stuff the kale, pepper, and almond cheese mixture into the pocket you created in each chicken breast. Pin the pocket closed with a toothpick to seal in the stuffing.
4. In a large bowl, mix the olive oil, cashew butter, lemon juice, and all spices and herbs until well combined.
5. Carefully dip the chicken breasts in this mixture one at a time, without allowing them to come unpinned. Make sure each breast is fully coated; it may be necessary to use your hands to spread the mixture onto the breasts to coat them evenly.
6. Grind the pistachios in a spice grinder or by hand with a mortar and pestle. Add to a large bowl along with the quinoa flakes, and dip each coated chicken breast into the crust mixture.
7. Heat the coconut oil in a large skillet over medium-high heat. Once the oil is melted, brown the chicken; this should take about a minute or two for each side.
8. Remove the chicken from the skillet, and place it in a glass baking dish.
9. Bake for 20 to 25 minutes, depending on the thickness of the chicken breast.

Adapted with permission from Dr. Mark Hyman's Chicken Breast Stuffed with Sun-Dried Tomato Pesto with Sautéed Spinach. Mark Hyman, *The Blood Sugar Solution 10-Day Detox Diet: Activate Your Body's Natural Ability to Burn Fat and Lose Weight Fast* (New York: Little Brown, 2014), p. 312.

## Cashew Cream Cheese

*Geek Out with Dr. Sara:* Soaking cashews in water reduces the amount of phytic acid in the nuts and aids in their digestion. Even though it has not yet sprouted, a soaked nut has begun its germination process and has released many of the same nutritious enzymes that are found in sprouts.

*Makes 4 to 6 servings*

  1 cup raw organic cashews, soaked in water overnight
  2 tablespoons full-fat unsweetened coconut milk
  Juice of one lemon
  1 teaspoon garlic salt
  ½ teaspoon black pepper
  3 tablespoons nutritional yeast

Blend all ingredients in a high-powered blender until smooth and creamy. Enjoy with celery sticks or sliced cucumbers.

## Spicy Mung Bean Hummus

Mung beans are not only easier to cook than other varieties of legumes; they are easier to digest as well. Since they don't have a tough outer layer, mung beans make for a quick, light, and creamy homemade hummus.

*Makes 4 to 6 servings*

  1 cup cooked mung beans
  Juice of one Meyer lemon
  ⅓ cup tahini

1 garlic clove
½ teaspoon harissa paste or ground cayenne pepper
½ teaspoon sea salt
¼ cup almond milk

Blend the mung beans, lemon juice, tahini, garlic, harissa or cayenne, and salt for several minutes in a blender or food processor. Slowly add the almond milk until the desired consistency is achieved. Serve with grain-free crackers or crudités.

Adapted with permission from Heidi Swanson's Mung Bean Hummus. Heidi Swanson, "Mung Bean Hummus Recipe," *101CookBooks.com*, accessed March 8, 2014, www .101cookbooks.com/archives/mung-bean-hummus-recipe.html.

## Creamy Dairy-Free Brie

*Makes 6 to 8 servings*

1 13-ounce can full-fat unsweetened coconut milk
1 tablespoon xanthan gum
1 tablespoon nutritional yeast
1 teaspoon salt
1 cup macadamia nuts, soaked overnight in water
Juice of one lemon

1. Bring the coconut milk to a boil in a medium saucepan, whisking frequently.
2. Reduce the heat to low, and stir in the xanthan gum, nutritional yeast, and ½ teaspoon salt. Whisk the mixture continuously for about a minute until thick.
3. Drain and rinse the macadamia nuts.
4. In a high-powered blender, combine the nuts, lemon juice, and 2 tablespoons of the warm coconut mixture. Blend until creamy and thick.
5. Line a small round cake pan or wooden cheese box with cheese-cloth, and spoon the macadamia mixture into a thick, even layer.

Mound the edges toward the center slightly so that the sides of the mixture are not touching the cloth.

6. Pour the remaining coconut mixture over the top, and smooth it into the channel you created around the edge so that a thin, even layer covers the top and sides of the cheese.

7. Cover loosely with cheese paper or the top of the wooden cheese box, and refrigerate overnight.

## THE HORMONE RESET DESSERTS

## Dr. Sara's Hormone Reset Brownies

*Geek Out with Dr. Sara:* A study of sweet potatoes in the *Journal of Nutrition and Metabolism* found that the way in which the potato is cooked will affect its glycemic index. Boiling was found to be the optimum cooking method for a lower glycemic index. The glycemic load in these grain-free brownies can be reduced further by substituting additional xylitol for coconut sugar.

*Makes 12 servings*

 2 medium sweet potatoes
 2 large eggs
 ½ cup organic, hardwood-derived xylitol
 ½ cup coconut sugar
 ½ cup avocado oil
 1 to 2 tablespoons sorghum flour
 1 tablespoon baking powder
 1 cup unsweetened pure cacao powder

*For the icing:*
 2 dark chocolate bars, 85 percent pure cacao or higher
 ¼ cup organic, hardwood-derived xylitol (adjust to taste)

1. Preheat the oven to 350°F.
2. Bring 6 cups water to a boil in a large pot.
3. Peel the sweet potatoes, and cut each into several large pieces. Add them to the boiling water, and cook until tender, approximately 30 minutes.
4. Strain the potatoes, and mash them with a fork in a large bowl.
5. Stir in the eggs, xylitol, coconut sugar, avocado oil, sorghum flour, baking powder, and cacao powder.
6. Pour batter into a greased 8 × 8-inch baking dish, and bake for 20 to 25 minutes.
7. Meanwhile, melt the chocolate bars in a microwave or double boiler. Stir the xylitol into the melted chocolate.
8. When the brownies are done, remove them from the oven, and pour the melted chocolate over the top to form a thin, even layer.
9. Allow the brownies to cool before serving.

## Chia Seed Pudding
..................................................................................................

*Geek Out with Dr. Sara:* Chia seeds contain substantial amounts of omega-3 fatty acids. Recent studies have shown omega-3s to increase insulin sensitivity, one of the underlying issues with regard to obesity and weight gain. In other words, this delicious dessert may actually help you lose weight!

*Makes 4 servings*

> ½ cup dry chia seeds
> 1 cup unsweetened coconut milk
> 1 teaspoon stevia powder

Place all ingredients in a jar or other glass container with a tight-fitting lid. Shake vigorously for 1 minute. Refrigerate for at least 2 hours, preferably overnight. Enjoy as a dessert or for breakfast.

## Almond Butter Fudge Bars

If you are not an almond butter fan, you can use cashew or macadamia nut butter instead in this dish. Be sure to find organic, unsweetened, cold-pressed almond butter. Most commercial almond butters are made from nuts that have been roasted at very high heat. Cold-pressed almond and other nut butters retain the vitamins and nutrients of the raw nut.

*Makes 8 to 10 servings*

> 3 large pure cacao or 100 percent dark chocolate bars (4 to 6 ounces each)
> 2 tablespoons coconut oil
> 2 teaspoons pure vanilla extract, divided
> 1½ cups organic, hardwood-derived xylitol, divided
> 1 cup full-fat canned coconut milk
> 1½ cups unsweetened almond butter

1. Break the chocolate bars into pieces, and melt them in a microwave or double boiler. Stir in the coconut oil, 1 teaspoon vanilla extract, and ½ cup xylitol.
2. Line a shallow baking dish with parchment paper, and pour the chocolate mixture into an even layer on the bottom of the dish. Place in the freezer for 30 minutes or until the chocolate has hardened.
3. Meanwhile, combine the rest of the xylitol and vanilla, the coconut milk, and the almond butter in a large bowl. Stir well.
4. Spread this mixture evenly over the hardened chocolate.
5. Cover, and freeze again for at least 1 hour. Cut into small squares. Serve cold, directly from the freezer.

# Resources

For an updated list of resources, visit www.HormoneReset.com.

### Roll Call: Your Metabolic Hormones

*Estrogen*

- A group of hormones produced primarily in the ovaries to promote female characteristics such as menstruation, breast growth, and hip growth.
- Other sources of estrogen include adrenal glands and fat cells.
- Estrogen grows your hips and breasts; regulates menstruation; builds uterine lining to prepare for pregnancy; and keeps women lubricated, from joints to vagina.

*Insulin*

- Drives glucose into cells as fuel and deposits fat.
- Chronically high insulin increases estrogen (specifically estrone) and increases cells' resistance to insulin.

*Leptin*

- Regulates appetite, satiety, and adiponectin, which adjusts how you burn fat.

*Cortisol*

- The main stress hormone, member of the glucocorticoid family.

- Governs blood sugar, blood pressure, and immune function.
- Cortisol is produced in your adrenal glands under most conditions, stressful or otherwise.

*Thyroid*
- Essential to the smooth operation of hormone pathways.
- Adequate thyroid hormone is necessary to make pregnenolone from cholesterol, and then to further refine it into progesterone.
- Affects metabolism and energy, weight, mood

*Growth Hormone*
- Helps burn fat and gain lean muscle. Determines how much fat is deposited on your belly.

*Testosterone*
- One of the sex hormones belonging to the androgen family.
- Although it is often thought of as the male hormone, women need to have some testosterone in their bodies as well. The difference between men and women lies in the quantity of testosterone (men produce much higher quantities).
- Hormone of vitality and self-confidence
- Producing too much is the main reason for female infertility in this country.
- Also involved in sex drive; producing too little is linked to low libido in women and men.

*Adiponectin*
- Secreted by fat cells and adjusts how you burn fat.

*Ghrelin*
- Raises appetite in order to initiate eating.
- Acts in counterpart to leptin.
- Produced in stomach cells.

*Oxytocin*
- Both a hormone and a neurotransmitter, which means it acts as a brain chemical that transmits information from nerve to nerve.

- Called by some "the love hormone" because it increases in the blood with orgasm in both men and women.
- Oxytocin is also released when the cervix dilates, thereby augmenting labor, and when a woman's nipples are stimulated, which facilitates breast-feeding and promotes bonding between mother and baby.

*DHEA*

- Can convert into testosterone when needed; member of androgen family.
- Affects mood and sex drive.
- Too much DHEA has been associated with acne and depression in menopause.

*Melatonin*

- Regulates our sleep/wake cycle.
- Helps control the timing and release of female reproductive hormones.

### Preparing for the Hormone Reset

For the measurements in chapter 2, use the following websites for handy calculators:

- Waist-to-hip ratio: www.healthstatus.com/calculate/waist-to-hip-ratio
- Body mass index (BMI): www.bmi-calculator.net
- Waist-to-height ratio (WHtR): www.health-calc.com/body-composition/waist-to-height-ratio
- Basal metabolic rate (BMR): www.bmi-calculator.net/bmr-calculator or www.bmrcalculator.org

These are my favorite devices for measurement:

- Sleep: Fitbit, UP by Jawbone
- Blood pressure: Omron for wrist or upper arm, Panasonic for upper arm

- Blood sugar: TrueResult Blood Glucose Starter Kit, OneTouch Ultra
- Steps: Fitbit, UP by Jawbone, iPhone
- Body fat: Omron Fat Loss Monitor, Tanita Body Fat Monitor

To learn about ways to talk to your doctor about ordering tests, see page 334–35 in *The Hormone Cure.*

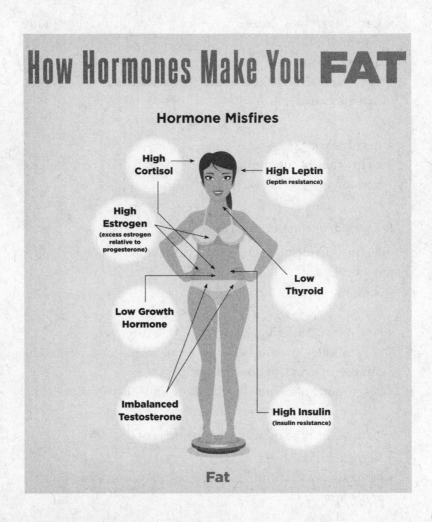

### Recommended Baseline Tests

*Estradiol level,* in blood or saliva, ideally performed on Day 3 or Day 21 if you're still menstruating regularly, and performed anytime if you're irregular or menopausal.

*Fasting glucose level,* drawn by lab personnel in a laboratory or measured with your own glucose meter and a finger stick.

*Fasting leptin level,* drawn by lab personnel in a laboratory.

*Morning cortisol level,* in blood or saliva.

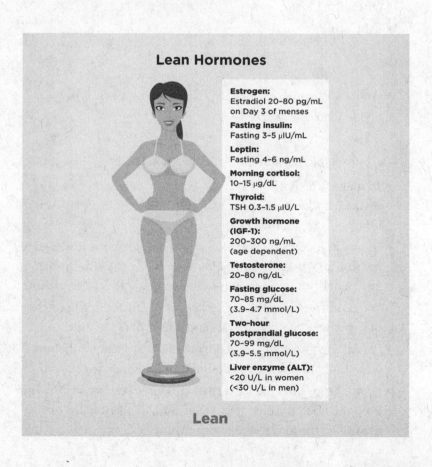

**Lean Hormones**

**Estrogen:**
Estradiol 20–80 pg/mL
on Day 3 of menses

**Fasting insulin:**
Fasting 3–5 µIU/mL

**Leptin:**
Fasting 4–6 ng/mL

**Morning cortisol:**
10–15 µg/dL

**Thyroid:**
TSH 0.3–1.5 µIU/L

**Growth hormone
(IGF-1):**
200–300 ng/mL
(age dependent)

**Testosterone:**
20–80 ng/dL

**Fasting glucose:**
70–85 mg/dL
(3.9–4.7 mmol/L)

**Two-hour
postprandial glucose:**
70–99 mg/dL
(3.9–5.5 mmol/L)

**Liver enzyme (ALT):**
<20 U/L in women
(<30 U/L in men)

**Lean**

*Thyroid panel,* including thyroid-stimulating hormone (TSH), free triiodothyronine (free T3, or FT3), and reverse triiodothyronine (reverse T3, or RT3).

*Growth hormone level,* typically measured in the blood as insulin-like growth factor 1 (IGF-1).

*Free testosterone level,* in blood or saliva.

### Recommended Laboratories

- Quest Diagnostics
- LabCorp
- Hunter Labs
- ZRTlab.com
- WellnessFx.com
- MyMedLab.com

### Resources for Maintaining Your Hormone Reset

- To make sure that your seafood is safe from mercury and other toxins, check out Seafood Watch by the Monterey Bay Aquarium: www.seafoodwatch.org.
- To find a shake that's compliant with the Hormone Reset, go to my store at www.DrGottfriedStore.com. I've personally formulated a delicious protein powder, fiber, and other supplements.
- For grain-free crackers, try flackers from Doctor in the Kitchen or dehydrated vegetable crackers from Lydia's Organics.
- For collagen—a source of clean protein—check out Bulletproof: www.bulletproofexec.com/bulletproof-upgraded-collagen/.
- For high-powered blenders that will purée your vegetables but keep the fiber, try Blendtec, Magic Bullet, NutriBullet, or Vitamix. I like the Magic Bullet for travel!

- For extra-dark chocolate, a few of my favorite organic brands are Dagoba organic chocolate; Sacred Chocolate, founded by health expert David Wolfe; and Tazo.
- I formulated a delicious bar that's compliant with the Hormone Reset. Find it at my online store: www.DrGottfriedStore.com.
- For coconut kefir, try Donna Gates's recipe: bodyecology.com /articles/secrets-for-making-perfect-young-coconut-kefir.php.

### Recommended Books

My first book is called *The Hormone Cure* (www.TheHormoneCure Book.com)

*Against All Grain* by Danielle Walker

*The Blood Sugar Solution 10-Day Detox Diet* by Mark Hyman

*The Disease Delusion* by Jeffrey Bland

*Good Calories, Bad Calories* by Gary Taubes

*The Paleo Approach* by Sarah Ballantyne

*Sugar Impact Diet, The Virgin Diet* and *The Virgin Diet Cookbook* by JJ Virgin

*WomanCode* by Alisa Vitti

*Your Personal Paleo Code* by Chris Kresser

# Acknowledgments

There are many people to thank for their contributions to this book, and not all of them are listed here. In particular, I want to acknowledge the following individuals.

My daughters, for enduring my love of writing and how it often competes for my attention

My parents, Albert and Mary Szal, for smiling gamely as I visited with the family in tow and spent most of the time with my nose in a book or laptop

My tireless mentor and dear friend, JJ Virgin

My agent, Celeste Fine, who took my complex protocols of how to reset metabolic hormones and organized them into a cohesive plan and who never seems to tire of my shenanigans

My dearest friends, especially Dr. Jo Ilfeld, for supporting me every step along the way and offering the most hilarious commentary as she read draft after draft of this book

My roommate from medical school, Dr. Meryl Rosofsky, M.D., and her beloved fiancé, Stuart Coleman—I am deeply indebted to you for invaluable support and life-altering questions over the years

My sisters, Anna and Justina, for their enduring support and dance parties

My best-kept secret, Leslie Murphy, for your endless energy and goodwill as you keep our family and home smoothly operating

My beloved readers, including Dr. Anna Cabeca, D.O.; Dr. Steven Masley, M.D.; Michael Lovitch; Robin Nielsen; Pattie Ptak; Lisa D. Schwab; Dr. Betty Suh-Burgmann, M.D.; Dr. Kat Toups, M.D.; and last but most important, my darling husband, David Gottfried

My former assistant, Dorianne Caswell, who expertly ran our test kitchen and cheerfully chauffeured my kids to volleyball and clarinet lessons

My patients, who have patiently waited while my writing and family duties took me away from their needs and deepest desires

My beta testers—about four thousand of you—who were the first to try out my protocol online, ask all the important questions, and track their progress and awesome successes: thank you!

My gifted editors, Nancy Hancock and Gideon Weil, at Harper-One—I'm so blessed to have worked with you. To my publisher, Mark Tauber, thank you for the gamble you took and for putting your skin in the game. To my publicist, Melinda Mullin, I felt you were simpatico when we first met. Warmest thanks to Laina Adler, vice president of marketing; Noël Chrisman and Terri Leonard for expert production; and Claudia Boutote, senior vice president and associate publisher.

My team: Rachel, my awesome assistant; Kenny Bushman, my tireless web guy; Kevin Plottner, my designer, who created all the illustrations in this book; Steven Kaufman, our superb general manager; Christina Wilson, our nutritionista. Biggest thanks to Brandi Abbey, Kelli Price, and Laura Friedlander for your unwavering support on the front lines at SaraGottfriedMD.com. Thanks also to Fanny Wilson for wrangling the cash flow!

My editors: Nora Isaacs and Elaine Hooker, I can't thank you enough for keeping the words true to my spirit and intentions

My podcast cohost: Huge thanks to Pedram Shojai, O.M.D., for taking us to number one on iTunes and reminding me to have more fun while working.

My colleagues and fellow warriors: Heartfelt thanks to Patrick Hanaway, M.D.; Cynthia Pasquella; Gary Taubes; Josh Axe, D.C.; Abel James; Dave Asprey; Alan Christianson, N.D.; Tom Malterre; Kevin Gianni; Nick Polizzi; and my favorite savant, Chris Kresser. I'm grateful to Sharon Melnick, Ph.D., for her unwavering support, introductions, and provocative questions. Humble pranams to Mark Hyman, M.D., for writing a stellar forward.

Most important, my greatest thanks to my husband, David Gottfried, who has supported me through thick and thin and who continues to be my greatest champion, confidant, and sounding board. I couldn't have written this book without your quirky humor, inspiration, relentless support, and loving encouragement.

I love you all.

# Notes

## Chapter 2: Prep for Your Hormone Reset

1. A. N. Gearhardt et al., "Preliminary Validation of the Yale Food Addiction Scale," *Appetite* 52, no. 2 (2009): 430–36, doi:10.1016/j.appet.2008.12.003; and A. J. Flint et al., "Food Addiction Scale Measurement in 2 Cohorts of Middle-Aged and Older Women," *American Journal of Clinical Nutrition* 99, no. 3 (2014): 578–86, doi:10.3945/ajcn.113.068965.
2. "Waist to Hip Ratio Calculator," University of Maryland Medical System, accessed March 8, 2014, www.healthcalculators.org/calculators/waist_hip.asp.
3. "Calculate Your Body Mass Index," National Heart Lung and Blood Institute, accessed March 8, 2014, www.nhlbi.nih.gov/guidelines/obesity/BMI/bmicalc.htm.
4. Here's a sample BMI calculation: "How to Calculate Your Body Mass Index (BMI)," WikiHow, accessed March 8, 2014, www.wikihow.com/Calculate-Your-Body-Mass-Index-(BMI). An alternative to BMI is ABSI, or A Body Shape Indicator. Learn more at absi.nl.eu.org.
5. L. M. Browning et al., "A Systematic Review of Waist-to-Height Ratio as a Screening Tool for the Prediction of Cardiovascular Disease and Diabetes: 0.5 Could Be a Suitable Global Boundary Value," *Nutrition Research Reviews* 23, no. 2 (2010): 247–69; and C. M. Lee et al., "Indices of Abdominal Obesity Are Better Discriminators of Cardiovascular Risk Factors than BMI: A Meta-Analysis," *Journal of Clinical Epidemiology* 61, no. 7 (2008): 646–53.
6. Here's an online calculator for waist-to-height ratio (WHtR): "Waist to Height Ratio," Health-calc, accessed March 14, 2014, www.health-calc.com/body-composition/waist-to-height-ratio.
7. Sara Gottfried, "Turn Your Insulin into Jillian Michaels (Part 1): Test Your Blood Sugar," Sara Gottfried, M.D., May 31, 2013, accessed March 11, 2014, www.saragottfriedmd.com/turn-your-insulin-into-jillian-michaels-part-1-test-your-blood-sugar/.
8. "Verified Products," Non-GMO Project, accessed December 12, 2014, www.nongmoproject.org/find-non-gmo/search-participating-products/.
9. M. Ball, "Want to Know If Your Food Is Genetically Modified?" *The Atlantic,* May 14, 2014, accessed June 14, 2014, www.theatlantic.com/features/archive/2014/05/want-to-know-if-your-food-is-genetically-modified/370812/.

10. B. López-González et al., "Association Between Magnesium-Deficient Status and Anthropometric and Clinical-Nutritional Parameters in Postmenopausal Women," *Nutrición Hospitalaria* 29, no. 3 (2014): 658–64.

## Chapter 3: Meatless

1. USDA Agricultural Research Service: National Agricultural Library, U.S. Department of Agriculture, accessed June 26, 2014, http://ndb.nal.usda.gov.
2. K. M. Flegal et al., "Prevalence of Obesity and Trends in the Distribution of Body Mass Index Among U.S. Adults 1999–2010," *Journal of the American Medical Association* 307, no. 5 (2012): 491–97; C. L. Ogden et al., "Prevalence of Overweight, Obesity, and Extreme Obesity Among Adults: United States, Trends 1960–1962 Through 2007–2008," *National Center for Health Statistics* 6 (2010): 1–6; and "Weight-Control Information Network: Overweight and Obesity Statistics," National Institute of Diabetes and Digestive Kidney Diseases, accessed June 22, 2014, http://win.niddk.nih.gov/statistics/.
3. P. E. Miller et al., "Dietary Patterns and Colorectal Adenoma and Cancer Risk: A Review of the Epidemiological Evidence," *Nutrition and Cancer* 62, no. 4 (2010): 413–24.
4. B. R. Goldin et al., "Estrogen Excretion Patterns and Plasma Levels in Vegetarian and Omnivorous Women," *New England Journal of Medicine* 307 (1982): 1542–47, doi:10.1056/NEJM198212163072502.
5. S. L. Gorbach et al., "Diet and the Excretion and Enterohepatic Cycling of Estrogens," *Preventative Medicine* 16, no. 4 (1987): 525–31.
6. "Superbugs Invade American Supermarkets," Environmental Working Group, accessed June 22, 2014, www.ewg.org/meateatersguide/superbugs/#sthash.GJnX2gbk.dpuf.
7. C. La Rocca et al., "From Environment to Food: The Case of PCB," *Annali dell'Istituto Superiore Di Sanità* 42, no. 4 (2006): 410–16; and R. Malisch et al., "Dioxins and PCBs in Feed and Food—Review from European Perspective," *Science of the Total Environment* (September 1, 2014), doi:10.1016/j.scitotenv.2014.03.022.
8. E. N. Ponnampalam et al., "Effect of Feeding Systems on Omega-3 Fatty Acids, Conjugated Linoleic Acid and Trans Fatty Acids in Australian Beef Cuts: Potential Impact on Human Health," *Asia Pacific Journal of Clinical Nutrition* 15, no. 1 (2006): 21–29; C. A. Daley et al., "A Review of Fatty Acid Profiles and Antioxidant Content in Grass-Fed and Grain-Fed Beef," *Nutrition Journal* 9, no. 1 (2010): 10, doi:10.1186/1475-2891-9-10; D. C. Rule et al., "Comparison of Muscle Fatty Acid Profiles and Cholesterol Concentrations of Bison, Beef Cattle, Elk, and Chicken," *Journal of Animal Science* 80, no. 5 (2002): 1202–11; S. K. Duckett et al., "Effects of Time on Feed on Beef Nutrient Composition," *Journal of Animal Science* 71, no. 8 (1993): 2079–88; K. Nuernberg et al., "Effect of a Grass-Based and a Concentrate Feeding System on Meat Quality Characteristics and Fatty Acid Composition of Longissimus Muscle in Different Cattle Breeds," *Livestock Production Science* 94, nos. 1–2 (2005): 137–47; and P. I. Ponte et al., "Influence of Pasture Intake on the Fatty Acid Composition, and Cholesterol, Tocopherols, and Tocotrienols Content in Meat from Free-Range Broilers," *Poultry Science* 87, no. 1 (2008): 80–88.
9. A. Pan et al., "Changes in Red Meat Consumption and Subsequent Risk of Type 2 Diabetes Mellitus: Three Cohorts of U.S. Men and Women," *JAMA Internal Medicine* 173, no. 14 (2013): 1328–35, doi:10.1001/jamainternmed.2013.6633.
10. R. Micha et al., "Red and Processed Meat Consumption and Risk of Incident Coronary Heart Disease, Stroke, and Diabetes Mellitus: A Systematic Review and Meta-Analysis," *Circulation* 121, no. 21 (2010): 2271–83.
11. J. A. Nettleton et al., "Dietary Patterns, Food Groups, and Telomere Length in the Multi-Ethnic Study of Atherosclerosis (MESA)," *American Journal of Clinical Nutrition* 88, no. 5 (2008): 1405–12; and Micha et al., "Red and Processed Meat Consumption," 2271–83.

12. N. Stettler et al., "Systematic Review of Clinical Studies Related to Pork Intake and Metabolic Syndrome or Its Components," *Diabetes, Metabolic Syndrome, and Obesity: Targets and Therapy* 6 (2013): 347–57.

13. C. De Filippo et al., "Impact of Diet in Shaping Gut Microbiota Revealed by a Comparative Study in Children from Europe and Rural Africa," *Proceedings of the National Academy of Sciences of the United States of America* 107, no. 33 (2010): 14691–96, doi:10.1073/pnas.1005963107; L. G. Albenberg et al., "Diet and the Intestinal Microbiome: Associations, Functions, and Implications for Health and Disease," *Gastroenterology* 146, no. 6 (2014): 1564–72, doi:10.1053/j.gastro.2014.01.058; and I. B. Jeffery et al., "Diet-Microbiota Interactions and Their Implications for Healthy Living," *Nutrients* 5, no. 1 (2013): 234–52, doi:10.3390/nu5010234.

14. R. E. Ley et al., "Microbial Ecology: Human Gut Microbes Associated with Obesity," *Nature* 444 (2006): 1022–23; and P. J. Turnbaugh et al., "An Obesity-Associated Gut Microbiome with Increased Capacity for Energy Harvest," *Nature* 444, no. 7122 (2006): 1027–131, doi:10.1038/nature05414.

15. Pew Commission on Industrial Farm Animal Production, the Pew Charitable Trusts and the Johns Hopkins Bloomberg School of Public Health, accessed June 7, 2014, www.ncifap.org/.

16. Nutritional data: Total calories: 1582 joules; total carbohydrates: 80 grams; total dietary fiber: 34 grams; net carbohydrates: 46 grams; total protein: 109 grams; total fat: 96 grams. For nutritional analysis wen consulted "Nutrition Facts," Self Nutrition Data, Condé Nast, accessed March 13, 2014, http://nutritiondata.self.com, and "Dr. Sara's Hormone Balancing Shakes (30 Servings)," Sara Gottfried, M.D., accessed March 12, 2014, https://pi127.infusionsoft.com/app/storeFront/showProductDetail?productId=332.

17. S. Reinwald et al., "Whole Versus the Piecemeal Approach to Evaluating Soy," *Journal of Nutrition* 140, no. 12 (2010): 2335S–43S, doi:10.3945/jn.110.124925.

18. R. Sapbamrer et al., "Effects of Dietary Traditional Fermented Soybean on Reproductive Hormones, Lipids, and Glucose Among Postmenopausal Women in Northern Thailand," *Asia Pacific Journal of Clinical Nutrition* 22, no. 2 (2013): 222–28, doi:10.6133/apjcn.2013.22.2.17.

19. Rick Hanson, *Hardwiring Happiness: The New Brain Science of Contentment, Calm, and Confidence* (New York: Harmony, 2013).

20 M. Heger et al., "Efficacy and Safety of a Special Extract of Rheum rhaponticum (ERr 731) in Perimenopausal Women with Climacteric Complaints: A 12-week Randomized, Double-blind, Placebo-Controlled Trial," *Menopause* 13, no. 5 (2006): 744–59; M. Kaszkin-Bettag et al., "The Special Extract ERr 731 of the Roots of Rheum rhaponticum Decreases Anxiety and Improves Health State and General Well-Being in Perimenopausal Women," *Menopause* 14, no. 2 (2007): 270–83; M. Kaszkin-Bettag et al., "Efficacy of the Special Extract ERr 731 from Rhapontic Rhubarb for Menopausal Complaints: A 6-month Open Observational Study," *Alternative Therapies in Health and Medicine* 14, no. 6 (2008): 32–38; M. Kaszkin-Bettag et al., "Confirmation of the Efficacy of ERr 731 in Perimenopausal Women with Menopausal Symptoms, " *Alternative Therapies in Health and Medicine* 15, no. 1 (2009): 24–34; and I. Hasper et al., "Long-Term Efficacy and Safety of the Special Extract ERr 731 of Rheum rhaponticum in Perimenopausal Women with Menopausal Symptoms," *Menopause* 16, no. 1 (2009): 117–31.

21. T. Yates et al., "Self-Reported Sitting Time and Markers of Inflammation, Insulin Resistance, and Adiposity," *American Journal of Preventative Medicine* 42, no. 1 (2012): 1–7, doi:10.1016/j.amepre.2011.09.022; and "No Hard Workouts Necessary to Avoid Diabetes—Just Cut Your Sitting Time by 90 Minutes a Day: Study," *NY Daily News*, March 4, 2013, www.nydailynews.com/life-style/health/hard-workouts-avoid-diabetes-sit-study-article-1.1278791.

## Chapter 4: Sugar Free

1. T. P. Markovic et al., "The Determinances of Glycemic Response to Diet Restrictions and Weight Loss in Obesity and NIDDM," *Diabetes Care* 21, no. 5 (1998): 687.
2. R. N. Smith et al., "The Effect of a High-Protein, Low Glycemic-Load Diet Versus a Conventional, High Glycemic-Load Diet on Biochemical Parameters Associated with Acne Vulgaris: A Randomized, Investigator-Masked, Controlled Trial," *Journal of the American Academy of Dermatology* 57, no. 2 (2007): 247–56.
3. R. Smith et al., "A Pilot Study to Determine the Short-Term Effects of a Low Glycemic Load Diet on Hormonal Markers of Acne: A Nonrandomized, Parallel, Controlled Feeding Trial," *Molecular Nutrition and Food Research* 52, no. 6 (2008): 718–26, doi:10.1002/mnfr.200700307.
4. P. Pedram et al., "Food Addiction: Its Prevalence and Significant Association with Obesity in the General Population," *PLoS ONE* 8, no. 9 (2013): e74832, doi:10.1371/journal.pone.0074832.
5. A. J. Flint et al., "Food-Addiction Scale Measurement in 2 Cohorts of Middle-Aged and Older Women," *American Journal of Clinical Nutrition* 99, no. 3 (2014): 578–86, doi:10.3945/ajcn.113.068965.
6. Judith Orloff, *Emotional Freedom* (New York: Random House, 2010).
7. N. M. Avena et al., "Evidence for Sugar Addiction: Behavioral and Neurochemical Effects of Intermittent, Excessive Sugar Intake," *Neuroscience and Biobehavioral Reviews* 32, no. 1 (2008): 20–39, doi:10.1016/j.neubiorev.2007.04.019; N. M. Avena et al., "Animal Models of Sugar and Fat Bingeing: Relationship to Food Addiction and Increased Body Weight," *Methods in Molecular Biology* 829 (2012): 351–65, doi:10.1007/978-1-61779-458-2_23; T. Ventura et al., "Neurobiologic Basis of Craving for Carbohydrates," *Nutrition* 30, no. 3 (2014): 252–56, doi:10.1016/j.nut.2013.06.010; and A. Hone-Blanchet et al., "Overlap of Food Addiction and Substance Use Disorders Definitions: Analysis of Animal and Human Studies," *Neuropharmacology* 85C (2014): 81–90, doi:10.1016/j.neuropharm.2014.05.019.
8. J. A. Schroeder et al., "Nucleus Accumbens C-Fos Expression Is Correlated with Conditioned Place Preference to Cocaine, Morphine, and High Fat/Sugar Food Consumption" (presentation, Connecticut College, New London, CT, November 13, 2013).
9. C. Imperatori et al., "The Association Among Food Addiction, Binge Eating Severity and Psychopathology in Obese and Overweight Patients Attending Low-Energy-Diet Therapy," *Comprehensive Psychiatry* (May 6, 2014), doi:10.1016/j.comppsych.2014.04.023.
10. M. Lenoir et al., "Intense Sweetness Surpasses Cocaine Reward," *PLoS ONE* 2, no. 8 (2007): e698, doi:10.1371/journal.pone.0000698.
11. M. Monachese et al., "Bioremediation and Tolerance of Humans to Heavy Metals Through Microbial Processes: A Potential Role for Probiotics?" *Applied and Environmental Microbiology* 78, no. 18 (2012): 6397–404, doi:10.1128/AEM.01665-12.
12. I. H. Choi et al., "Kimchi, a Fermented Vegetable, Improves Serum Lipid Profiles in Healthy Young Adults: Randomized Clinical Trial," *Journal of Medicinal Food* 16, no. 3 (2013): 223–29, doi:10.1089/jmf.2012.2563.
13. Nutritional data: Total calories: 1700 joules; total carbohydrates: 51 grams; total dietary fiber: 19; net carbohydrates: 32 grams; total protein: 122 grams; total fat: 114 grams. For nutritional analysis, we consulted the following: "Nutrition Facts," Self Nutrition Data, Condé Nast, accessed March 11, 2014, http://nutritiondata.self.com; Gord Kerr, "Ghee Nutrition Information," Livestrong, August 16, 2013, accessed March 12, 2014, www.livestrong.com/article/363779-ghee-nutrition-information; and "Basic Report: 05664, Ground Turkey, Fat Free, Patties, Broiled," Agricultural Research Service, U.S. Department of Agriculture, accessed March 12, 2014, http://ndb.nal.usda.gov/ndb/foods/show/1089?fg=&man=&lfacet=&count=&max=25&qlookup=ground+turkey

&offset=&sort=&format=Abridged&reportfmt=other&rptfrm=&ndbno=&nutrient1=
&nutrient2=&nutrient3=&subset=&totCount=&measureby=&_action_show=Apply+
Changes&Qv=1&Q2586=1.0&Q2587=6.0, and "Dr. Sara's Hormone Balancing Shakes
(30 Servings)," Sara Gottfried M.D., accessed March 12, 2014, https://pi127.infusionsoft
.com/app/storeFront/showProductDetail?productId=332.

## Chapter 5: Fruitless

1. N. Wiebe et al., "A Systematic Review on the Effect of Sweeteners on Glycemic Response
and Clinically Relevant Outcomes," *BMC Medicine* 9 (2011): 123, doi:10.1186/1741-
7015-9-123; and L. M. Hanover et al., "Manufacturing, Composition, and Application
of Fructose," *American Journal of Clinical Nutrition* 58, suppl. 5 (1993): 724S–32S.

2. R. H. Lustig, "Fructose: It's 'Alcohol Without the Buzz,'" *Advances in Nutrition* 4, no.
2 (2013): 226–35; R. H. Lustig, *Fat Chance: Beating the Odds Against Sugar, Processed
Food, Obesity, and Disease* (New York: Hudson Street Press, 2012); and G. A. Bray et al.,
"Dietary Sugar and Body Weight: Have We Reached a Crisis in the Epidemic of Obesity
and Diabetes?: Health Be Damned! Pour on the Sugar," *Diabetes Care* 37, no. 4 (2014):
950–56, doi:10.2337/dc13-2085.

3. D. Faeh et al., "Effect of Fructose Overfeeding and Fish Oil Administration on Hepatic
De Novo Lipogenesis and Insulin Sensitivity in Healthy Men," *Diabetes* 54, no. 7 (2005):
1907–13; and V. Lecoultre et al., "Effects of Fructose and Glucose Overfeeding on
Hepatic Insulin Sensitivity and Intrahepatic Lipids in Healthy Humans," *Obesity (Silver
Spring)* 21, no. 4 (2013): 782–85, doi:10.1002/oby.20377.

4. M. Dirlewanger et al., "Effects of Fructose on Hepatic Glucose Metabolism in Humans,"
*American Journal of Physiology, Endocrinology, and Metabolism* 279, no. 4 (2000): E907–11;
Y. Wei et al., "Hepatospecific Effects of Fructose on C-Jun NH2-Terminal Kinase: Impli-
cations for Hepatic Insulin Resistance," *American Journal of Physiology, Endocrinology, and
Metabolism* 287, no. 5 (2004): E926–33; K. L. Stanhope et al., "Consuming Fructose-
Sweetened, Not Glucose-Sweetened, Beverages Increases Visceral Adiposity and Lipids
and Decreases Insulin Sensitivity in Overweight/Obese Humans," *Journal of Clinical
Investigation* 119, no. 5 (2009): 1322–34; and L. Tappy et al., "Metabolic Effects of
Fructose and the Worldwide Increase in Obesity," *Physiological Reviews* 90, no. 1 (2010):
23–46, doi:10.1152/physrev.00019.2009.

5. J. R. Vasselli et al., "Dietary Components in the Development of Leptin Resistance,"
*Advances in Nutrition* 4, no. 2 (2013): 164–75, doi:10.3945/an.112.003152; and M.
Aijälä et al., "Long-Term Fructose Feeding Changes the Expression of Leptin Receptors
and Autophagy Genes in the Adipose Tissue and Liver of Male Rats: A Possible Link
to Elevated Triglycerides," *Genes and Nutrition* 8, no. 6 (2013): 623–35, doi:10.1007/
s12263-013-0357-3.

6. S. E. Lakhan et al., "The Emerging Role of Dietary Fructose in Obesity and Cognitive
Decline," *Nutrition Journal* 12 (2013): 114, doi:10.1186/1475-2891-12-114; A. P. Simo-
poulos, "Dietary Omega-3 Fatty Acid Deficiency and High Fructose Intake in the Devel-
opment of Metabolic Syndrome, Brain Metabolic Abnormalities, and Non-Alcoholic
Fatty Liver Disease," *Nutrients* 5, no. 8 (2013): 2901–23, doi:10.3390/nu5082901; and
R. Agrawal et al., "'Metabolic Syndrome' in the Brain: Deficiency in Omega-3 Fatty
Acid Exacerbates Dysfunctions in Insulin Receptor Signalling and Cognition," *Journal
of Physiology* 590, pt. 10 (2012): 2485–99.

7. "Profiling Food Consumption in America," Agriculture Fact Book, USDA, accessed
June 25, 2014, www.usda.gov/factbook/chapter2.pdf.

8. "USDA National Nutrient Database for Standard Reference," Agricultural Research
Service, National Agricultural Library, USDA, accessed June 26, 2014, http://ndb.nal
.usda.gov.

9. M. B. Vos et al., "Dietary Fructose Consumption Among U.S. Children and Adults: The Third National Health and Nutrition Examination Survey," *Medscape Journal of Medicine* 10, no. 7 (2008): 160.

10. B. C. Fam et al., "The Liver: Key in Regulating Appetite and Body Weight," *Adipocyte* 1, no. 4 (2012): 259–64.

11. H. K. Gonnissen et al., "Chronobiology, Endocrinology, and Energy- and Food-Reward Homeostasis," *Obesity Reviews* 14, no. 5 (2013): 405–16, doi:10.1111/obr.12019.

12. A. Liu et al., "Habitual Shortened Sleep and Insulin Resistance: An Independent Relationship in Obese Individuals," *Metabolism: Clinical and Experimental* 62, no. 11 (2013): 1553–56, doi:10.1016/j.metabol.2013.06.003; and A. Liu et al., "Risk for Obstructive Sleep Apnea in Obese, Nondiabetic Adults Varies with Insulin Resistance Status," *Sleep and Breathing* 17, no. 1 (2013): 333–38, doi:10.1007/s11325-012-0696-0.

13. R. R. Markwald et al., "Impact of Insufficient Sleep on Total Daily Energy Expenditure, Food Intake, and Weight Gain," Proceedings of the National Academy of Sciences of the United States of America 110, no. 14 (2013): 5695–700, doi:10.1073/pnas.1216951110.

14. L. F. Lien et al., "The STEDMAN Project: Biophysical, Biochemical, and Metabolic Effects of a Behavioral Weight Loss Intervention During Weight Loss, Maintenance, and Regain," *OMICS* 13, no. 1 (2009): 21–35, doi:10.1089/omi.2008.0035.

15. M. R. Carnethon et al., "Association of Weight Status with Mortality in Adults with Incident Diabetes," *Journal of the American Medical Association* 308, no. 6 (2012): 581–90, doi:10.1001/jama.2012.9282.

16. Calculate your body fat percentage on their website. "Percentage Body Fat Calculator: Skinfold Method," American Council on Exercise, accessed September 23, 2013, http://www.acefitness.org/acefit/healthy_living_tools_content.aspx?id=2.

17. R. V. Considine et al., "Serum Immunoreactive-Leptin Concentrations in Normal-Weight and Obese Humans," *New England Journal of Medicine* 334, no. 5 (1996): 292–95.

18. P. R. Gibson et al., "Evidence-Based Dietary Management of Functional Gastrointestinal Symptoms: The FODMAP Approach," *Journal of Gastroenterology and Hepatology* 25, no. 2 (2010): 252–58, doi:10.1111/j.1440-1746.2009.06149.x.

19. J. Ratliff et al., "Carbohydrate Restriction (With or Without Additional Dietary Cholesterol Provided by Eggs) Reduces Insulin Resistance and Plasma Leptin Without Modifying Appetite Hormones in Adult Men," *Nutrition Research* 29, no. 4 (2009): 262–68, doi:10.1016/j.nutres.2009.03.007.

20. Nutritional data: Total calories: 1475 joules; total carbohydrates: 82 grams; total dietary fiber: 35 grams; net carbohydrates: 47 grams; total protein: 97 grams; total fat: 86 grams. For nutritional analysis, we consulted "Nutrition Facts," Self Nutrition Data, Condé Nast, accessed March 13, 2014, http://nutritiondata.self.com, and "Dr. Sara's Hormone Balancing Shakes (30 Servings)," Sara Gottfried, M.D., accessed March 12, 2014, https://pi127.infusionsoft.com/app/storeFront/showProductDetail?productId=332.

21. Agrawal et al., "'Metabolic Syndrome' in the Brain," 2485–99; A. P. Ross et al., "A High Fructose Diet Impairs Spatial Memory in Male Rats," *Neurobiology of Learning and Memory* 92, no. 3 (2009): 410–16; D. A. Costello et al., "Brain Deletion of Insulin Receptor Substrate 2 Disrupts Hippocampal Synaptic Plasticity and Metaplasticity," *PLoS ONE* 7, no. 2 (2012): e31124; and M. Hariri et al., "Does Omega-3 Fatty Acids Supplementation Affect Circulating Leptin Levels? A Systematic Review and Meta-Analysis on Randomized Controlled Clinical Trials," *Clinical Endocrinology* (May 24, 2014), doi:10.1111/cen.12508.

22. J. M. Tishinsky, "Modulation of Adipokines by n-3 Polyunsaturated Fatty Acids and Ensuing Changes in Skeletal Muscle Metabolic Response and Inflammation," *Applied Physiology, Nutrition, and Metabolism* 38, no. 3 (2013): 361, doi:10.1139/apnm-2012-0447; M. J. Moreno-Aliaga et al., "Regulation of Adipokine Secretion by n-3 Fatty Acids," *Proceedings of the Nutrition Society* 69, no. 3 (2010): 324–32, doi:10.1017/S0029665110001801; and M. Mostowik et al., "Omega-3 Polyunsaturated Fatty Acids

NOTES **305**

Increase Plasma Adiponectin to Leptin Ratio in Stable Coronary Artery Disease," *Cardiovascular Drugs and Therapy* 27, no. 4 (2013): 289–95, doi:10.1007/s10557-013-6457-x.

23. L. S. Baylor et al., "Resting Thyroid and Leptin Hormone Changes in Women Following Intense, Prolonged Exercise Training," *European Journal of Applied Physiology* 88, nos. 4–5 (2003): 480–84; and R. R. Kraemer et al., "Serum Leptin Concentrations in Response to Acute Exercise in Postmenopausal Women With and Without Hormone Replacement Therapy," *Proceedings of the Society for Experimental Biology and Medicine* 221, no. 3 (1999): 171–77.

## Chapter 6: Caffeine Free

1. O. G. Cameron et al., "Caffeine and Human Cerebral Blood Flow: A Positron Emission Tomography Study," *Life Sciences* 47, no. 13 (1990): 1141–46; A. Nehlig et al., "Caffeine and the Central Nervous System: Mechanisms of Action, Biochemical, Metabolic, and Psychostimulant Effects," *Brain Research Reviews* 17, no. 2 (1992): 139–70; A. S. Field et al., "Dietary Caffeine Consumption and Withdrawal: Confounding Variables in Quantitative Cerebral Perfusion Studies?" *Radiology* 227, no. 1 (2003): 129–35; M. J. Lunt et al., "Comparison of Caffeine-Induced Changes in Cerebral Blood Flow and Middle Cerebral Artery Blood Velocity Shows That Caffeine Reduces Middle Cerebral Artery Diameter," *Physiological Measurement* 25, no. 2 (2004): 467–74; and M. A. Addicott et al., "The Effect of Daily Caffeine Use on Cerebral Blood Flow: How Much Caffeine Can We Tolerate?" *Human Brain Mapping* 30, no. 10 (2009): 3102–14, doi:10.1002/hbm.20732.
2. M. al'Absi et al., "Hypothalamic-Pituitary-Adrenocortical Responses to Psychological Stress and Caffeine in Men at High and Low Risk for Hypertension," *Psychosomatic Medicine* 60, no. 4 (1998): 521–27.
3. R. Corti et al., "Coffee Acutely Increases Sympathetic Nerve Activity and Blood Pressure Independently of Caffeine Content: Role of Habitual Versus Nonhabitual Drinking," *Circulation* 106, no. 23 (2002): 2935–40.
4. "Stress by Gender: A Stressful Imbalance," American Psychological Association, accessed September 9, 2013, www.apa.org/news/press/releases/stress/2012/gender.aspx.
5. T. C. Adam et al., "Stress, Eating, and the Reward System," *Physiology and Behavior* 91, no. 4 (2007): 449–58; and E. S. Epel, "Psychological and Metabolic Stress: A Recipe for Accelerated Cellular Aging?" *Hormones (Athens)* 8, no. 1 (2009): 7–22.
6. J. Dauhenmier et al., "Changes in Stress, Eating, and Metabolic Factors Are Related to Changes in Telomerase Activity in a Randomized Mindfulness Intervention Pilot Study," *Psychoneuroendocrinology* 37, no. 7 (2012): 917–28, doi:10.1016/j.psyneuen.2011.10.008.
7. Anahad O'Connor, "The Claim—A Person Can Pay Off a Sleep Debt by Sleeping Late on Weekends," *New York Times* online, November 2, 2009, accessed September 9, 2013, www.nytimes.com/2009/11/03/health/03real.html?_r=0.
8. K. Spiegel et al., "Effects of Poor and Short Sleep on Glucose Metabolism and Obesity Risk," *Nature Reviews Endocrinology* 5, no. 5 (2009): 253–61, doi:10.1038/nrendo.2009.23; and L. Morselli et al., "Role of Sleep Duration in the Regulation of Glucose Metabolism and Appetite," *Best Practice and Research: Clinical Endocrinology and Metabolism* 24, no. 5 (2010): 687–702, doi:10.1016/j.beem.2010.07.005.
9. S. R. Patel et al., "Association Between Reduced Sleep and Weight Gain in Women," *American Journal of Epidemiology* 164, no. 10 (2006): 947–54.
10. See Gregg Jacobs's column: Gregg D. Jacobs, Ph.D., "10 Tips to Better Sleep," MedHelp, December 16, 2008, accessed March 11, 2014, www.medhelp.org/user_journals/show/47782/10-tips-to-better-sleep.
11. D. J. Wallis et al., "Emotions and Eating: Self-Reported and Experimentally Induced Changes in Food Intake Under Stress," *Appetite* 52, no. 2 (2009): 355–62.
12. N. J. Nevanperä et al., "Occupational Burnout, Eating Behavior, and Weight Among Work-

ing Women," *American Journal of Clinical Nutrition* 95, no. 4 (2012): 934–43, doi:10.3945/ajcn.111.014191.

13. Nutritional data: Total calories: 1848 joules; total carbohydrates: 91 grams; total dietary fiber: 43 grams; net carbohydrates: 48 grams; total protein: 116 grams; total fat: 119 grams. For nutritional analysis, we consulted "Nutrition Facts," Self Nutrition Data, Condé Nast, accessed March 13, 2014, http://nutritiondata.self.com, and "Dr. Sara's Hormone Balancing Shakes (30 Servings)," Sara Gottfried, M.D., accessed March 12, 2014, https://pi127.infusionsoft.com/app/storeFront/showProductDetail?productId=332.

14. J. N. McClintick et al., "Stress-Response Pathways Are Altered in the Hippocampus of Chronic Alcoholics," *Alcohol* 47, no. 7 (2013): 505–15, doi:10.1016/j.alcohol.2013.07.002.

15. R. Hursel et al., "Green Tea Catechin Plus Caffeine Supplementation to a High-Protein Diet Has No Additional Effect on Body Weight Maintenance After Weight Loss," *American Journal of Clinical Nutrition* 89, no. 3 (2009): 822–30.

16. I. A. Hakim et al., "Preparation, Composition and Consumption Patterns of Tea-Based Beverages in Arizona," *Nutrition Research* 20, no 12 (2000): 1715–24.

17. J. D. Lambert et al., "Dose-Dependent Levels of Epigallocatechin-3-Gallate in Human Colon Cancer Cells and Mouse Plasma and Tissues," *Drug Metabolism and Disposition* 34, no. 1 (2006):8–11.

18. M. C. Venables et al., "Green Tea Extract Ingestion, Fat Oxidation, and Glucose Tolerance in Healthy Humans," *American Journal of Clinical Nutrition* 87 (2008): 778–84; and Y. Fukino et al., "Randomized Controlled Trial for an Effect of Green Tea-Extract Powder Supplementation on Glucose Abnormalities," *European Journal of Clinical Nutrition* 62, no. 8 (2008): 953–60.

19. L. Hartley et al., "Green and Black Tea for the Primary Prevention of Cardiovascular Disease," *Cochrane Database of Systematic Reviews* (June 18, 2013): 6:CD009934. doi: 10.1002/14651858.CD009934.pub2.

20. T. M. Jurgens et al., "Can Green Tea Preparations Help with Weight Loss?" *Canadian Pharmacists Journal (Ottawa)* 147, no. 3 (2014): 159-60; T. M. Jurgens et al., "Green Tea for Weight Loss and Weight Maintenance in Overweight or Obese Adults," *Cochrane Database of Systematic Reviews* (December 12, 2012) 12:CD008650. doi: 10.1002/14651858 .CD008650.pub2; and A. Basu et al., "Green Tea Supplementation Affects Body Weight, Lipids, and Lipid Peroxidation in Obese Subjects with Metabolic Syndrome," *Journal of the American College of Nutrition* 29, no. 1 (2010): 31–40.

21. Donald Lee Goss, "A Comparison of Lower Extremity Joint Work and Initial Loading Rates Among Four Different Running Styles" (Ph.D. dissertation, University of North Carolina at Chapel Hill, 2012), ChiRunning, accessed March 6, 2014, www.chirunning .com/2012%20UNC%20Running%20Impact%20Study.pdf.

22. T. Kino, "Circadian Rhythms of Glucocorticoid Hormone Actions in Target Tissues: Potential Clinical Implications," *Science Signaling* 5, no. 244 (2012): pt4, doi:10.1126/scisignal.2003333.

## Chapter 7: Grain Free

1. Gena Lee Nolin and Mary Shomon, *Beautiful Inside and Out: Conquering Thyroid Disease with a Healthy, Happy, "Thyroid Sexy" Life* (New York: Atria, 2013).

2. P. K. Crane et al., "Glucose Levels and Risk of Dementia," *New England Journal of Medicine* 369, no. 6 (2013): 540–48, doi:10.1056/NEJMoa1215740.

3. Y. Hu et al., "Dietary Glycemic Load, Glycemic Index, and Associated Factors in a Multiethnic Cohort of Midlife Women," *Journal of the American College of Nutrition* 28, no. 6 (2009): 636–47; S. Oba et al., "Dietary Glycemic Index, Glycemic Load, and

Intake of Carbohydrate and Rice in Relation to Risk of Mortality from Stroke and Its Subtypes in Japanese Men and Women," *Metabolism* 59, no. 11 (2010): 1574–82; S. Liu et al., "Relation Between a Diet with a High Glycemic Load and Plasma Concentrations of High-Sensitivity C-Reactive Protein in Middle-Aged Women," *American Journal of Clinical Nutrition* 75, no. 3 (2002): 492–98; and K. Murakami et al., "Associations of Dietary Glycaemic Index and Glycaemic Load with Food and Nutrient Intake and General and Central Obesity in British Adults," *British Journal of Nutrition* 110, no. 11 (2013): 2047–57, doi:10.1017/S0007114513001414.

4. D. Yu et al., "Dietary Carbohydrates, Refined Grains, Glycemic Load, and Risk of Coronary Heart Disease in Chinese Adults," *American Journal of Epidemiology* 178, no. 10 (2013): 1542–49, doi:10.1093/aje/kwt178.

5. J. E. Chavarro et al., "A Prospective Study of Dietary Carbohydrate Quantity and Quality in Relation to Risk of Ovulatory Infertility," *European Journal of Clinical Nutrition* 63, no. 1 (2009): 78–86, doi:10.1038/sj.ejcn.1602904.

6. T. L. Halton et al., "Low-Carbohydrate-Diet Score and the Risk of Coronary Heart Disease in Women," *New England Journal of Medicine* 355, no. 19 (2006): 1991–2002, doi:10.1056/NEJMoa055317.

7. S. Liu et al., "Relation Between Changes in Intakes of Dietary Fiber and Grain Products and Changes in Weight and Development of Obesity Among Middle-Aged Women," *American Journal of Clinical Nutrition* 78, no. 5 (2003): 920–27.

8. "Number (in Millions) of Civilian, Noninstitutionalized Persons with Diagnosed Diabetes, United States, 1980–2011," Centers for Disease Control and Prevention, accessed February 4, 2014, www.cdc.gov/diabetes/statistics/prev/national/figpersons.htm.

9. Y. Rodriguez-Carrasco et al., "Exposure Estimates to Fusarium Mycotoxins Through Cereal Intake," *Chemosphere* 93, no. 10 (2013): 2297-303.

10. M. Ryberg et al., "A Palaeolithic-Type Diet Causes Strong Tissue-Specific Effects on Ectopic Fat Deposition in Obese Postmenopausal Women," *Journal of Internal Medicine* 274, no. 1 (2013): 67–76, doi:10.1111/joim.12048.

11. "The Top 5 Reasons Vitamin D Makes Women Bulletproof," Bulletproof, accessed March 6, 2014, www.bulletproofexec.com/the-top-5-reasons-vitamin-d-makes-women-bulletproof/.

12. I. Depoortere, "Taste Receptors of the Gut: Emerging Roles in Health and Disease," *Gut* 63, no. 1 (2014): 179–90, doi:10.1136/gutjnl-2013-305112; and S. C. Kinnamon, "Neurosensory Transmission Without a Synapse: New Perspectives on Taste Signaling," *BMC Biology* 11 (2013): 42, doi:10.1186/1741-7007-11-42.

13. A. Sapone et al., "Divergence of Gut Permeability and Mucosal Immune Gene Expression in Two Gluten-Associated Conditions: Celiac Disease and Gluten Sensitivity," *BMC Medicine* 9 (2011): 23, doi:10.1186/1741-7015-9-23.

14. Angela Haupt, "Are Gluten-Free Cosmetics Necessary?" *U.S. News and World Report*, September 11, 2012, accessed March 12, 2014, http://health.usnews.com/health-news/articles/2012/09/11/are-gluten-free-cosmetics-necessary; and Kate Murphy, "Jury Is Still Out on Gluten, the Latest Dietary Villian," *New York Times* online, May 8, 2007, accessed January 28, 2014, www.nytimes.com/2007/05/08/health/08glut.html.

15. Stephanie Strom, "A Big Bet on Gluten-Free," *New York Times* online, February 17, 2014, accessed March 12, 2014, www.nytimes.com/2014/02/18/business/food-industry-wagers-big-on-gluten-free.html?_r=1; Kate Murphy, "Jury Is Still Out on Gluten, the Latest Dietary Villian," *New York Times* online, May 8, 2007, accessed January 28, 2014, www.nytimes.com/2007/05/08/health/08glut.html; A. Tammaro et al., "Cutaneous Hypersensitivity to Gluten," *Dermatitis* 23, no. 5 (2012): 220–21; Y. Chinuki et al., "Higher Allergenicity of High Molecular Weight Hydrolysed Wheat Protein in Cosmetics for Percutaneous Sensitization," *Contact Dermatitis* 68, no. 2 (2013): 86–93, doi:10.1111/

j.1600-0536.2012.02168.x; and Shivani Vora, "Going Without Gluten," *New York Times* online, May 29, 2013, accessed January 28, 2014, www.nytimes.com/2013/05/30/fashion /going-without-gluten-beauty-spots.html.

16. Keith O'Brien, "Should We All Go Gluten-Free?" *New York Times* online, November 25, 2011, accessed January 28, 2014, www.nytimes.com/2011/11/27/magazine/Should-We-All-Go-Gluten-Free.html?pagewanted=all&_r=0.

17. C. Catassi et al., "Non-Celiac Gluten Sensitivity: The New Frontier of Gluten Related Disorders," *Nutrients* 5, no. 10 (2013): 3839–53, doi:10.3390/nu5103839.

18. P. D. Mooney et al., "Non-Celiac Gluten Sensitivity: Clinical Relevance and Recommendations for Future Research," *Neurogastroenterology and Motility* 25, no. 11 (2013): 864–71, doi:10.1111/nmo.12216.

19. Kristina Campbell, "Metaflora: *Wheat Belly* Book Review," Intestinal Gardener, December 29, 2012, accessed January 28, 2014, http://intestinalgardener.blogspot. com/2012/12/metaflora-wheat-belly-book-review.html.

20. Anya Sacharow, "What's Your Wheat Problem?" *Time* online, January 23, 2013, accessed January 28, 2014, http://ideas.time.com/2013/01/23/whats-your-wheat-problem/.

21. Loren Cordain, "Cereal Grains: Humanity's Double-Edged Sword," Department of Exercise and Sport Science, Colorado State University, accessed March 6, 2014, www .direct-ms.org/pdf/EvolutionPaleolithic/Cereal%20Sword.pdf.

22. T. Jönsson et al., "Agrarian Diet and Diseases of Affluence—Do Evolutionary Novel Dietary Lectins Cause Leptin Resistance?" *BMC Endocrine Disorders* 5, no. 10 (2005), doi:10.1186/1472-6823-5-10.

23. M. N. Akçay et al., "The Presence of the Antigliadin Antibodies in Autoimmune Thyroid Diseases," *Hepatogastroenterology* 50, suppl. 2 (2003): cclxxix–cclxxx.

24. Nutritional data: Total calories: 1546 joules; total carbohydrates: 71 grams; total dietary fiber: 23 grams; net carbohydrates: 48 grams; total protein: 108 grams; total fat: 102 grams. For nutritional analysis, we consulted the following: "Nutrition Facts," Self Nutrition Data, Condé Nast, accessed March 12, 2014, http://nutritiondata.self.com; "Dr. Sara's Hormone Balancing Shakes (30 Servings)," Sara Gottfried, M.D., accessed March 12, 2014, https://pi127.infusionsoft.com/app/storeFront/showProductDetail? productId=332; and "Basic Report: 19904, Chocolate, Dark, 70–85% Cacao Solids," Agricultural Research Service, U.S. Department of Agriculture, accessed March 12, 2014, http://ndb.nal.usda.gov/ndb/foods/show/6337?fg=&man=&lfacet=&count=& max=25&qlookup=cacao&offset=&sort=&format=Abridged&reportfmt=other&rptf rm=&ndbno=&nutrient1=&nutrient2=&nutrient3=&subset=&totCount=&measure by=&_action_show=Apply+Changes&Qv=0.15&Q12136=1.0&Q12137=1.0.

25. S. Kayaniyil et al., "Prospective Associations of Vitamin D with ß-Cell Function and Glycemia: The PROspective Metabolism and Islet Cell Evaluation (PROMISE) Cohort Study," *Diabetes* 60, no. 11 (2011): 2947–53; and C. Gagnon et al., "Low Serum 25-Hydroxyvitamin D Is Associated with Increased Risk of the Development of the Metabolic Syndrome at Five Years: Results from a National, Population-Based Prospective Study (The Australian Diabetes, Obesity, and Lifestyle Study: AusDiab)," *Journal of Clinical Endocrinology and Metabolism* 97, no. 6 (2012): 1953–61.

26. T. Christiansen et al., "Comparable Reduction of the Visceral Adipose Tissue Depot After a Diet-Induced Weight Loss With or Without Aerobic Exercise in Obese Subjects: A 12-Week Randomized Intervention Study," *European Journal of Endocrinology* 160, no. 5 (2009): 759–67, doi:10.1530/EJE-08-1009.

27. I. Ismail et al., "A Systematic Review and Meta-Analysis of the Effect of Aerobic vs. Resistance Exercise Training on Visceral Fat," *Obesity Reviews* 13, no. 1 (2012): 68–91, doi:10.1111/j.1467-789X.2011.00931.x.

28. Gretchen Reynolds, "The Scientific 7-Minute Workout," *Well* (blog), *New York*

*Times* online, May 9, 2013, accessed January 28, 2014, http://well.blogs.nytimes.com/2013/05/09/the-scientific-7-minute-workout/?_r=0.

29. Gretchen Reynolds, "For a 7-Minute Workout, Try Our New App," *New York Times* online, accessed December 2, 2014, http://well.blogs.nytimes.com/2014/10/24/for-a-7-minute-workout-download-our-new-app/.

## Chapter 8: Dairy Free

1. J. K. Jarvis et al., "Overcoming the Barrier of Lactose Intolerance to Reduce Health Disparities," *Journal of the National Medical Association* 94, no. 2 (2002): 55–66; "Lactose Intolerance Statistics," Statistic Brain, from the National Digestive Diseases Information Clearinghouse, accessed January 14, 2014, www.statisticbrain.com/lactose-intolerance-statistics/; and A. Høst, "Frequency of Cow's Milk Allergy in Childhood," *Annals of Allergy, Asthma, and Immunology* 89, no. 6, suppl. 1 (2002): 33–37, doi:10.1016/S1081-1206(10)62120-5.

2. D. P. Robinson et al., "Elevated 17ß-Estradiol Protects Females from Influenza A Virus Pathogenesis by Suppressing Inflammatory Responses," *PLoS Pathogens* 7, no. 7 (2011): e1002149, doi:10.1371/journal.ppat.1002149; and "Hormones and Oral Health," WebMD, accessed March 6, 2014, www.webmd.com/oral-health/hormones-oral-health.

3. D. Furman et al., "Systems Analysis of Sex Differences Reveals an Immunosuppressive Role for Testosterone in the Response to Influenza Vaccination," *Proceedings of the National Academy of Sciences of the United States of America* 111, no. 2 (2014): 869–74, doi:10.1073/pnas.1321060111; Brendan Maher, "Women Are More Vulnerable to Infections," *Nature* online, July 26, 2013, accessed March 6, 2014, www.nature.com/news/women-are-more-vulnerable-to-infections-1.13456; and "Arthritis: Frequently Asked Questions," Centers for Disease Control and Prevention, accessed March 6, 2014, www.cdc.gov/arthritis/basics/faqs.htm.

4. Kriss Carr, *Crazy Sexy Diet* (New York: Skirt, 2011): 34-36; personal communication with the author.

5. "Lactose Intolerance," Mayo Clinic, accessed January 28, 2014, www.mayoclinic.org/diseases-conditions/lactose-intolerance/basics/tests-diagnosis/CON-20027906; and "Lactose Tolerance Tests," Medline Plus, accessed January 28, 2014, www.nlm.nih.gov/medlineplus/ency/article/003500.htm.

6. L. C. Harrison et al., "Cow's Milk and Type 1 Diabetes: The Real Debate Is About Mucosal Immune Function," *Diabetes* 48, no. 8 (1999): 1501–7; and H. E. Wasmuth et al., "Cow's Milk and Immune-Mediated Diabetes," *Proceedings of the Nutrition Society* 59, no. 4 (2000): 573–79.

7. D. W. Niebuhr et al., "Association Between Bovine Casein Antibody and New Onset Schizophrenia Among U.S. Military Personnel," *Schizophrenia Research* 128, nos. 1–3 (2011): 51–55, doi:10.1016/j.schres.2011.02.005.

8. Jane E. Brody, "Personal Health; You Are Also What You Drink," *New York Times* online, March 27, 2007, accessed January 28, 2014, http://query.nytimes.com/gst/fullpage.html?res=990DE3D61230F934A15750C0A9619C8B63.

9. Sara Gottfried, "Kicking the Dairy Habit," Sara Gottfried, M.D., June 16, 2012, accessed January 14, 2014, www.saragottfriedmd.com/kicking-the-dairy-habit-why-its-so-friggin-hard-plus-several-tips-to-get-er-done/.

10. Sara Gottfried, "How I Fixed My Exercise, Got Lean, and Rocked My Growth Hormone (IGF-1)," Sara Gottfried, M.D., March 20, 2014, www.saragottfriedmd.com/biohacking-exercise-dose-exercise-rocked-growth-hormone/.

11. David Barboza, "Monsanto Sues Dairy in Maine Over Label's Remarks on Hormones," *New York Times* online, July 12, 2003, accessed January 14, 2014, www.nytimes.com/

2003/07/12/business/monsanto-sues-dairy-in-maine-over-label-s-remarks-on-hormones.html.

12. Andrew Pollack, "Maker Warns of Scarcity of Hormone for Dairy Cows," *New York Times* online, January 27, 2004, accessed January 14, 2014, www.nytimes.com/2004/01/27/business/maker-warns-of-scarcity-of-hormone-for-dairy-cows.html.

13. Nutritional data: Total calories: 1643 joules; total carbohydrates: 76 grams; total dietary fiber: 28 grams; net carbohydrates: 48 grams; total protein: 123 grams; total fat: 98 grams. For nutritional analysis, we consulted "Nutrition Facts," Self Nutrition Data, Condé Nast, accessed March 12, 2014, http://nutritiondata.self.com, and "Dr. Sara's Hormone Balancing Shakes (30 Servings)," Sara Gottfried, M.D., accessed March 12, 2014, https://pi127.infusionsoft.com/app/storeFront/showProductDetail?productId=332.

14. Save money by making coconut kefir at home. Check out the YouTube video.

15. "Lactase Chewable Tablets," Drugs.com, accessed January 28, 2014, www.drugs.com/cdi/lactase-chewable-tablets.html.

16. A. C. Utter et al., "Influence of Diet and/or Exercise on Body Composition and Cardiorespiratory Fitness in Obese Women," *International Journal of Sport Nutrition* 8, no. 3 (1998): 213–22.

17. T. Sijie et al., "High Intensity Interval Exercise Training in Overweight Young Women," *Journal of Sports Medicine and Physical Fitness* 52, no. 3 (2012): 255–62.

18. K. S. Weston et al., "High-Intensity Interval Training in Patients with Lifestyle-Induced Cardiometabolic Disease: A Systematic Review and Meta-Analysis," *British Journal of Sports Medicine* (October 21, 2013), doi:10.1136/bjsports-2013-092576.

19. Sara Gottfried, "How I Fixed My Exercise, Got Lean, and Rocked My Growth Hormone (IGF-1)," Sara Gottfried, M.D., March 20, 2014, www.saragottfriedmd.com/biohacking-exercise-dose-exercise-rocked-growth-hormone/.

20. "Sprint 8 FAQ," Vision Fitness, accessed January 28, 2014, www.visionfitness.com/content/sprint-8-faq.

## Chapter 9: Toxin Free

1. Maureen Rice, "Revealed . . . the 515 Chemicals Women Put on Their Bodies Every Day," *Daily Mail Online*, November 20, 2009, accessed March 6, 2014, www.dailymail.co.uk/femail/beauty/article-1229275/Revealed--515-chemicals-women-bodies-day.html.

2. K. S. Kim et al., "Interaction Between Persistent Organic Pollutants and C-Reactive Protein in Estimating Insulin Resistance Among Non-Diabetic Adults," *Journal of Preventative Medicine and Public Health* 45, no. 2 (2012): 62–69, doi:10.3961/jpmph.2012.45.2.62; L. Lind et al., "Can Persistent Organic Pollutants and Plastic-Associated Chemicals Cause Cardiovascular Disease?" *Journal of Internal Medicine* 271, no. 6 (2012): 537–53, doi:10.1111/j.1365-2796.2012.02536.x; R. T. Zoeller et al., "Endocrine-Disrupting Chemicals and Public Health Protection: A Statement of Principles from the Endocrine Society," *Endocrinology* 153, no. 9 (2012): 4097–110, doi:10.1210/en.2012-1422; D. H. Lee et al., "Association Between Serum Concentrations of Persistent Organic Pollutants and Insulin Resistance Among Nondiabetic Adults: Results from the National Health and Nutrition Examination Survey 1999–2002," *Diabetes Care* 30, no. 3 (2007): 622–28; J. Li et al., "Effects of Chronic Exposure to DDT and TCDD on Disease Activity in Murine Systemic Lupus Erythematosus," *Lupus* 18, no. 11 (2009): 941–49, doi:10.1177/0961203309104431; P. Langer, "The Impacts of Organochlorines and Other Persistent Pollutants on Thyroid and Metabolic Health," *Frontiers in Neuroendocrinology* 31, no. 4 (2010): 497–518, doi:10.1016/j.yfrne.2010.08.001; and V. Roos et al., "Circulating Levels of Persistent Organic Pollutants in Relation to Visceral and Subcutaneous Adipose Tissue by Abdominal MRI," *Obesity (Silver Spring, MD)* 21, no. 2 (2013): 413–18, doi:10.1002/oby.20267.

3. P. M. Lind et al., "Circulating Levels of Persistent Organic Pollutants Are Related to Retrospective Assessment of Life-Time Weight Change," *Chemosphere* 90, no. 3 (2013): 998–1004, doi:10.1016/j.chemosphere.2012.07.051.

4. B. J. Davis et al., "Di-(2-ethylhexyl) Phthalate Suppresses Estradiol and Ovulation in Cycling Rats," *Toxicology and Applied Pharmacology* 128 (1994): 216–223; T. Lovekamp-Swan et al., "Mechanisms of Phthalate Ester Toxicity in the Female Reproductive System," *Environmental Health Perspectives* 111, no. 2 (2003): 139–45; C. Richter et al., "Estradiol and Bisphenol A Stimulate Androgen Receptor and Estrogen Receptor Gene Expression in Fetal Mouse Prostate Mesenchyme Cells," *Environmental Health Perspectives* 115 (2007): 902–8; G. S. Prins, "Endocrine Disruptors and Prostate Cancer Risk." *Endocrine-Related Cancer,* 15 (2008): 649–56. C. Frizzell et al, "Endocrine Disrupting Effects of Zearalenone, Alpha- and Beta-zearalenol at the Level of Nuclear Receptor Binding and Steroidogenesis," *Toxicology Letters* 206, no. 2 (2011): 210–7; C. Teng et al., "Bisphenol A Affects Androgen Receptor Function via Multiple Mechanisms," *Chemico-Biological Interactions* 203, no. 3 (2013): 556–64; C. Frizzell et al., "Effects of the Mycotoxin Patulin at the Level of Nuclear Receptor Transcriptional Activity and Steroidogenesis in Vitro," *Toxicology Letters* 229, no. 2 (2014): 366–73.

5. E. Diamanti-Kandarakis et al., "Phenotypes and Environmental Factors: Their Influence in PCOS," *Current Pharmaceutical Design* 18, no. 3 (2012): 270–82; L. Akin et al., "The Endocrine Disruptor Bisphenol A May Play a Role in the Aetiopathogenesis of Polycystic Ovary Syndrome in Adolescent Girls," *Acta Paediatrica* Dec 3, 2014 doi: 10.1111/apa.12885.

6. L. Dodds, "Synthetic Oestrogenic Agents without the Phenanthrene Nucleus," *Nature* 137 (1936): 996; H. J. Lee et al., "Antiandrogenic Effects of Bisphenol A and Nonylphenol on the Function of Androgen Receptor," *Toxicological Sciences* 75, no. 1 (2003): 40–6; C. Teng et al., "Bisphenol A Affects Androgen Receptor Function via Multiple Mechanisms," *Chemico-Biological Interactions* 203, no. 3 (2013): 556–64; P. Fenichel et al., "Bisphenol A: An Endocrine and Metabolic Disruptor," *Annales d'endocrinologie* (Paris) 74, no. 3 (2013): 211–20; M. Ronn et al., "Bisphenol A Is Related to Circulating Levels of Adiponectin, Leptin and Ghrelin, but Not to Fat Mass or Fat Distribution in Humans," *Chemosphere* 112 (2014): 42–8; L. Le Corre et al., "BPA, an Energy Balance Disruptor," *Critical Reviews in Food Science and Nutrition* 55, no. 6 (2015): 769–77.

7. "Endocrine Disruptors," National Institute of Environmental Health Sciences, National Institutes of Health, May 2010, accessed January 28, 2014, www.niehs.nih.gov/health/materials/endocrine_disruptors_508.pdf.

8. L. Patrick, "Thyroid Disruption: Mechanisms and Clinical Implications in Human Health," *Alternative Medicine Review* 14, no. 4 (2009): 326–46.

9. J. D. Meeker et al., "Relationship Between Urinary Phthalate and Bisphenol A Concentrations and Serum Thyroid Measures in U.S. Adults and Adolescents from the National Health and Nutrition Examination Survey (NHANES) 2007–2008," *Environmental Health Perspectives* 119, no. 10 (2011): 1396–1402, doi:10.1289/ehp.1103582.

10. L. Dodds, "Synthetic Oestrogenic Agents without the Phenanthrene Nucleus," *Nature* 137 (1936): 996; H. J. Lee et al., "Antiandrogenic Effects of Bisphenol A and Nonylphenol on the Function of Androgen Receptor," *Toxicological Sciences* 75, no. 1 (2003): 40–6; C. Teng et al., "Bisphenol A Affects Androgen Receptor Function via Multiple Mechanisms," *Chemico-Biological Interactions* 203, no. 3 (2013): 556–64; P. Fenichel et al., "Bisphenol A: An Endocrine and Metabolic Disruptor," *Annales d'endocrinologie* (Paris) 74, no. 3 (2013): 211–20; M. Ronn et al., "Bisphenol A Is Related to Circulating Levels of Adiponectin, Leptin and Ghrelin, but Not to Fat Mass or Fat Distribution in Humans," *Chemosphere* 112 (2014): 42–8; L. Le Corre et al., "BPA, an Energy Balance Disruptor," *Critical Reviews in Food Science and Nutrition* 55, no. 6 (2015): 769–77.

11. R. J. Jandacek et al., "Reduction of the Body Burden of PCBs and DDE by Dietary

Intervention in a Randomized Trial," *Journal of Nutritional Biochemistry* 25, no. 4 (2014): 483–88.

12. Y. Ingenbleek et al., "Nutritional Essentiality of Sulfur in Health and Disease," *Nutrition Reviews* 71, no. 7 (2013): 413–32, doi:10.1111/nure.12050; and M. E. Nimni et al., "Are We Getting Enough Sulfur in Our Diet?" *Nutrition and Metabolism (London)* 4 (2007): 24.

13. Chris Kresser has an excellent series of articles on his blog about salt: Chris Kresser, "Shaking Up the Salt Myth: Healthy Salt Recommendations," *Chris Kresser* (blog), accessed March 13, 2014, http://chriskresser.com/shaking-up-the-salt-myth-healthy-salt-recommendations.

14. Nutritional data: Total calories: 1835 joules; total carbohydrates: 96 grams; total dietary fiber: 48 grams; net carbohydrates: 48 grams; total protein: 79 grams; total fat: 123 grams. For nutritional analysis, we consulted the following: "Nutritional Information," PopSugar, accessed March 13, 2014, www.fitsugar.com/latest/nutritional-information; "Basic Report: 19904, Chocolate, dark, 70–85% cacao solids," Agricultural Research Service, U.S. Department of Agriculture, accessed March 13, 2014, http://ndb.nal.usda .gov/ndb/foods/show/6337?fg=&man=&lfacet=&format=&count=&max=25&offset= &sort=&qlookup=cacao; "Nutrition Facts," Self Nutrition Data, Condé Nast, accessed March 13, 2014, http://nutritiondata.self.com; and "Dr. Sara's Hormone Balancing Shakes (30 Servings)," Sara Gottfried, M.D., accessed March 12, 2014, https://pi127 .infusionsoft.com/app/storeFront/showProductDetail?productId=332.

15. "The Nitty Gritty of Filter Types and Technologies," Environmental Working Group, February 27, 2013, accessed January 28, 2014, www.ewg.org/report/ewgs-water-filter-buying-guide/filter-technology.

## Chapter 10: Reentry

1. Rick Hanson and Richard Mendius, *Buddha's Brain: The Practical Neuroscience of Happiness, Love, and Wisdom* (Oakland: New Harbinger, 2009).

2. Susan Seliger, "'Superfoods' Everyone Needs," WebMD, accessed March 3, 2014, www .webmd.com/diet/features/superfoods-everyone-needs.

3. Nutritional data: Total calories: 1291 joules; total carbohydrates: 82 grams; total dietary fiber: 45 grams; net carbohydrates: 37; total protein: 79 grams; total fat: 77 grams. For nutritional analysis, we consulted the following: "Calories in Quinoa Flakes," SparkPeople, accessed March 13, 2014, www.sparkpeople.com/calories-in .asp?food=quinoa+flakes; "Nutrition Facts," Self NutritionData, Condé Nast, accessed March 13, 2014, http://nutritiondata.self.com, and "Dr. Sara's Hormone Balancing Shakes (30 Servings)," Sara Gottfried, M.D., accessed March 12, 2014, https://pi127 .infusionsoft.com/app/storeFront/showProductDetail?productId=332.

4. J. Yin et al., "Efficacy of Berberine in Patients with Type 2 Diabetes Mellitus," *Metabolism: Clinical and Experimental* 57, no. 5 (2008): 712–17, doi:10.1016/j.metabol.2008.01.013.

5. Stephanie Chandler, "Toxicity and Berberine HCL Supplements," Livestrong, last modified February 19, 2014, www.livestrong.com/article/547840-toxicity-and-berberine-hcl-supplements/.

## Chapter 11: Sustenance

1. P. I. Sumithran et al., "The Defence of Body Weight: A Physiological Basis for Weight Regain After Weight Loss," *Clinical Science (London)* 124, no. 4 (2013): 231–41, doi:10.1042 /CS20120223; B. Richelsen et al., "Why Is Weight Loss So Often Followed by Weight Regain? Basal Biological Response as a Possible Explanation," *Ugeskrift for Laeger*, 168 no. 2 (2006): 159–63. [Article in Danish]

2. K. I. Johansson et al., "Effects of Anti-Obesity Drugs, Diet, and Exercise on Weight-Loss Maintenance After a Very-Low-Calorie Diet or Low-Calorie Diet: A Systematic Review

and Meta-Analysis of Randomized Controlled Trials," *American Journal of Clinical Nutrition* 99, no. 1 (2014): 14–23, doi:10.3945/ajcn.113.070052; E. A. Martens et al., "Protein Diets, Body Weight Loss and Weight Maintenance," *Current Opinion in Clinical Nutrition and Metabolic Care* 17, no. 1 (2014): 75–79, doi:10.1097/MCO.0000000000000006; M. S. Westerterp-Plantenga et al., "Dietary Protein: Its Role in Satiety, Energetics, Weight Loss and Health," *British Journal of Nutrition* 108 (2012): Suppl 2:S105–12, doi:10.1017/S0007114512002589; M. P. I. Lejeune et al., "Additional Protein Intake Limits Weight Regain After Weight Loss in Humans," *British Journal of Nutrition* 93, no. 2 (2005): 281–89; M. S. Westerterp-Plantenga et al., "High Protein Intake Sustains Weight Maintenance After Body Weight Loss in Humans," *International Journal of Obesity and other Related Metabolic Disorders* 28, no. 1 (2014): 57–64.

3. L. Schwingshackl et al., "Long-Term Effects of Low Glycemic Index/Load vs. High Glycemic Index/Load Diets on Parameters of Obesity and Obesity-Associated Risks: A Systematic Review and Meta-Analysis," *Nutrition, Metabolism, and Cardiovascular diseases* 23, no. 8 (2013): 699–706, doi:10.1016/j.numecd.2013.04.008.

4. S. Phelan et al., "Are the Eating and Exercise Habits of Successful Weight Losers Changing?" *Obesity (Silver Spring)* 14, no. 4 (2006): 710–16.

5. H. M. Niemeier et al., "Internal Disinhibition Predicts Weight Regain Following Weight Loss and Weight Loss Maintenance," *Obesity (Silver Spring)* 15, no. 10 (2007): 2485–94. From Niemeier's work, two factors affected weight loss maintenance: (1) an "internal" factor that described eating in response to internal cues, such as feelings and thoughts; and (2) an "external" factor that described eating in response to external cues, such as social events. When you have more internal disinhibition, you're at greater risk of poor weight loss outcomes.

6. S. Berkemeyer, "Acid-Base Balance and Weight Gain: Are There Crucial Links via Protein and Organic Acids in Understanding Obesity?" *Medical Hypotheses* 73, no. 3 (2009): 347–56. doi:10.1016/j.mehy.2008.09.059.1.

7. R. K. Edwards et al., "The Association of Maternal Obesity with Fetal pH and Base Deficit at Cesarean Delivery," *Obstetrics and Gynecology* 122, no. 2, pt. 1 (2013): 262–67, doi:10.1097/AOG.0b013e31829b1e62.

8. L. M. Donini et al., "How to Estimate Fat Mass in Overweight and Obese Subjects," *International Journal of Endocrinology* (2013): 2856–80, doi:10.1155/2013/285680.

9. H. K. Gonnissen et al., "Sleep Architecture When Sleeping at an Unusual Circadian Time and Associations with Insulin Sensitivity," *PLoS One* 8, no. 8 (2013): e72877, doi:10.1371/journal.pone.0072877; H. K. Gonnissen et al., "Chronobiology, Endocrinology, and Energy- and Food-Reward Homeostasis," *Obesity Reviews* 14, no.5 (2013): 405–16; T. Roenneberg et al., "Social Jetlag and Obesity," *Current Biology* 22 (2012): 939–43, doi:10.1016/j.cub.2012.03.038; S. M. Hampton et al., "Postprandial Hormone and Metabolic Responses in Simulated Shift Work," *Journal of Endocrinology* 151 (1996): 259–67, doi:10.1677/joe.0.1510259; F. A. Scheer et al., "Adverse Metabolic and Cardiovascular Consequences of Circadian Misalignment," *Proceedings of the National Academy of Sciences of the United States of America* 106 (2009): 4453–58, doi:10.1073/pnas.0808180106; H. K. Gonnissen et al., "Effect of a Phase Advance and Phase Delay of the 24-h Cycle on Energy Metabolism, Appetite, and Related Hormones," *American Journal of Clinical Nutrition* 96 (2012): 689–97, doi:10.3945/ajcn.112.037192; and F. Rutters et al., "Distinct Associations Between Energy Balance and the Sleep Characteristics Slow Wave Sleep and Rapid Eye Movement Sleep," *International Journal of Obesity* 36 (2012): 1346–52, doi:10.1038/ijo.2011.250.

10. J. G. Thomas et al., "Weight-Loss Maintenance for 10 Years in the National Weight Control Registry," *American Journal of Preventative Medicine* 46, no. 1 (2014): 17–23, doi:10.1016/j.amepre.2013.08.019; R. R. Wing et al., "Long-Term Weight Loss Maintenance," *American Journal of Clinical Nutrition* 82 (1 Suppl) (2005): 222S–25S.

11. L. G. Ogden et al., "Cluster Analysis of the National Weight Control Registry to Identify Distinct Subgroups Maintaining Successful Weight Loss," *Obesity (Silver Spring)* 20, no. 10 (2012): 2039–47, doi:10.1038/oby.2012.79.

12. V. A. Catenacci et al., "Dietary Habits and Weight Maintenance Success in High Versus Low Exercisers in the National Weight Control Registry," *Journal of Physical Activity and Health* (2013), PMID: 24385447 [epub ahead of print].

13. S. Phelan et al., "Empirical Evaluation of Physical Activity Recommendations for Weight Control in Women," *Medicine and Science in Sports and Exercise* 39, no. 10 (2007): 1832–36. Findings support current recommendations that more activity may be needed to prevent weight regain than to prevent weight gain. Including some higher-intensity activity may also be advisable for weight-loss maintenance.

14. V. A. Catenacci et al., "Physical Activity Patterns Using Accelerometry in the National Weight Control Registry," *Obesity (Silver Spring)* 19, no. 6 (2011): 1163–70, doi:10.1038/oby.2010.264.

15. V. A. Catenacci et al., "Dietary Habits and Weight Maintenance Success in High Versus Low Exercisers in the National Weight Control Registry," *Journal of Physical Activity and Health* (December 31, 2013) [epub ahead of print].

16. "Is It Possible to Care Too Much? Understanding How to Care Without It Becoming a Source of Your Stress," HeartMath, accessed March 4, 2014, www.heartmath.com/articles/overcare-article.html.

17. Billy Graham, *The Holy Spirit: Activating God's Power in Your Life,* (Thomas Nelson: Nashville, TN 1978), 92. The Christian's inner struggle is as follows: "An Eskimo fisherman came to town every Saturday afternoon. He always brought his two dogs with him. One was white and the other was black. He had taught them to fight on command. Every Saturday afternoon in the town square the people would gather and these two dogs would fight and the fisherman would take bets. On one Saturday, the black dog would win; another Saturday the white dog would win—but the fisherman always won! His friends began to ask him how he did it. He said, "I starve one and feed the other. The one I feed always wins because he is stronger.""

# Index

taste buds, 156
Tea and Collagen Frappe, 261
telomere care system, 129
testosterone, 80, 288
testosterone reset: *see* toxin free (testosterone reset)
tests: *see* baseline laboratory tests
Thai Coconut Chicken Soup (Tom Kha Gai), 267–68
thyroid, 288
thyroid disease, 157, 162
thyroid disruptors, 200
thyroid panel, 292
thyroid reset: *see* grain free (thyroid reset)
tomatoes, 116, 225
tongue scraper, 37
toxin free (testosterone reset), 195–215; beauty products and, 202–4; case files, 197–98; cell to soul practice, 211–12; exercise, 212–13; expectations when detoxing, 209–10; metabolism blockers, 199–202; micronutrients and, 204–5; mitochondria and, 202; notes from hormone resetters, 214; overview, 195–96; rules, 206–7; sample menu, 208; science behind, 198–99; self-assessment, 196–97; supplements, 210; testing, 213–14; water filters and, 207–9
toxins, 154
treadmill desks, 71
triglycerides, 241
Tulsi tea, 258–59
turkey, 38, 225
TV watching, 247
tyrosine, 92

vegan diet, 49
vegan foods, 187
vegetable oils, 39

vegetables, 38, 53–54, 89, 109, 156, 164–65, 206, 225
vinegar, 39
vitamin D, 155, 167

waist and hips measurement, 25–27, 244, 289
waist-to-height ratio measurement, 289
waist-to-height ratio (WHtR), 28
walnuts, 39, 62, 90, 225
water, 40, 71
Watercress and Arugula Salad with Green Goddess Dressing, 263–64
water filters, 207–9
weight gain, 10–12, 57, 84, 129–30, 154, 198, 244
weight loss strategies, 246–47
weight regain, 240
weight retention, 57
Weight Watchers diet, 4
wheat belly, 159, 160–61
whey, 180–81
*Why Do I Still Have Thyroid Symptoms?* (Kharrazian), 162
wild game, 49, 58, 155, 230
Wolfe, David, 204
worry, 211–12

xenobiotics, 199
xenoestrogen (fake estrogen), 203

yoga, 119, 138, 195, 211, 212–13, 251
yoga breathing, 169
yoga cleansing practices, 212–13
yoga poses, 138, 139
yogurt, 90, 106, 186, 225

Zucchini Noodles with Arugula Pesto, 271–72

# About the Author

Sara Gottfried, M.D., is the *New York Times* bestselling author of *The Hormone Cure*. After graduating from the physician-scientist training program at Harvard Medical School and MIT, Dr. Gottfried completed her residency at the University of California at San Francisco. She is a board-certified gynecologist who teaches natural hormone balancing in her novel online programs so that women can lose weight, detoxify, and feel great. Dr. Gottfried lives in Berkeley, California, with her husband and two daughters.

"An effective, easy-to-follow plan to balance your hormones and become lean, energetic, and loving life again. Stop settling and reclaim your sexy!"

—JJ Virgin, nutritionist and fitness expert, author of *The Virgin Diet* and *JJ Virgin's Sugar Impact Diet*

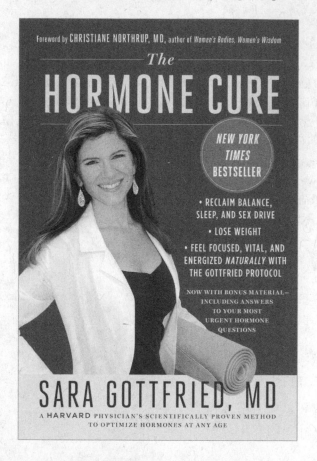

AVAILABLE FROM 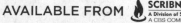  SCRIBNER
A Division of Simon & Schuster
A CBS COMPANY